Pharmacology

NOTICE

Medicine is an ever-changing science. As new research and clinical experience broaden our knowledge, changes in treatment and drug therapy are required. The editors and the publisher of this work have made every effort to ensure that the drug dosage schedules herein are accurate and in accord with the standards accepted at the time of publication. Readers are advised, however, to check the product information sheet included in the package of each drug they plan to administer to be certain that changes have not been made in the recommended dose or in the contraindications for administration. This recommendation is of particular importance in regard to new or infrequently used drugs.

Pharmacology:
PreTest® Self-Assessment and Review

Third Edition

Edited by

Priscilla S. Dannies, Ph.D.
Associate Professor of Pharmacology
Yale University School of Medicine
New Haven, Connecticut

John W. Kozarich, Ph.D.
Associate Professor of Pharmacology
Yale University School of Medicine
New Haven, Connecticut

John Stephen Lazo, Ph.D.
Assistant Professor of Pharmacology
Yale University School of Medicine
New Haven, Connecticut

McGraw-Hill Book Company
Health Professions Division
PreTest Series

New York St. Louis San Francisco Auckland Bogotá Guatemala Hamburg Johannesburg Lisbon London Madrid Mexico Montreal New Delhi Panama Paris Saõ Paulo Singapore Sydney Tokyo Toronto

Library of Congress Cataloging in Publication Data
Main entry under title:

Pharmacology : PreTest self-assessment and review.

Rev. ed. of: Pharmacology / edited by Robert E. Humphreys . . . [et al.]. 2nd ed. c1980.
Bibliography: p.
1. Pharmacology—Examinations, questions, etc.
I. Dannies, Priscilla S. II. Kozarich, John W.
III. Lazo, John S. [DNLM: 1. Pharmacology—Examination questions. QV 18 P5365]
RM300.P52 1983 615'.1'076 82-20321

ISBN 0-07-051935-8

Editor: *John H. Gilchrist*
Project Editor: *Merla C. Davies*
Editorial Assistant: *Donna Altieri*
Production: *Rosemary J. Pascale, Judith M. Raccio*
Designer: *Robert Tutsky*
Printer: *Hull Printing Company*

2 3 4 5 6 7 8 9 HUHU 8 7 6 5 4 3

Contents

List of Contributors

Kristin R. Carlson, Ph.D.
Associate Professor of Pharmacology
University of Massachusetts Medical School
Worcester, Massachusetts

Priscilla S. Dannies, Ph.D.
Associate Professor of Pharmacology
Yale University School of Medicine
New Haven, Connecticut

Robert E. Humphreys, M.D., Ph.D.
Associate Professor of Pharmacology and Medicine
University of Massachusetts Medical School
Worcester, Massachusetts

John W. Kozarich, Ph.D.
Associate Professor of Pharmacology
Yale University School of Medicine
New Haven, Connecticut

John Stephen Lazo, Ph.D.
Assistant Professor of Pharmacology
Yale University School of Medicine
New Haven, Connecticut

M. G. Marinus, Ph.D.
Associate Professor of Pharmacology
University of Massachusetts Medical School
Worcester, Massachusetts

Emil R. Smith, Ph.D.
Associate Professor of Pharmacology
University of Massachusetts Medical School
Worcester, Massachusetts

Introduction

Pharmacology: PreTest® Self-Assessment and Review has been designed to provide medical students, as well as physicians, with a comprehensive and convenient instrument for self-assessment and review. The 500 questions provided have been designed to parallel the format and degree of difficulty of the questions contained in Part I of the National Board of Medical Examiners examinations, the Federation Licensing Examination (FLEX), the Visa Qualifying Examination, and the ECFMG examination.

Each question in the book is accompanied by an answer, a paragraph explanation, and a specific page reference to either a current journal article, a textbook, or both. A bibliography, listing all the sources used in the book, follows the last chapter.

Perhaps the most effective way to use this book is to allow yourself one minute to answer each question in a given chapter; as you proceed, indicate your answer beside each question. By following this suggestion, you will be approximating the time limits imposed by the board examinations previously mentioned.

When you finish answering the questions in a chapter, you should then spend as much time as you need verifying your answers and carefully reading the explanations. Although you should pay special attention to the explanations for the questions you answered incorrectly, you should read **every** explanation. The contributors to this book have designed the explanations to reinforce and supplement the information tested by the questions. If, after reading the explanations for a given chapter, you feel you need still more information about the material covered, you should consult and study the references indicated.

This book meets the criteria established by the AMA's Department of Continuing Medical Education for up to 22 hours of credit in category 5D for the Physician's Recognition Award. It should provide an experience that is instructive as well as evaluative; we also hope that you enjoy it. We would be very happy to receive your comments.

General Principles

DIRECTIONS: Each question below contains five suggested answers. Choose the **one best** response to each question.

1. On the assumption that passive transport of the nonionized forms of the following drugs determines the rate of their absorption, which of the following drugs will be best absorbed in the small intestine?

(A) Acetylsalicylic acid, pK_a 3.0
(B) Boric acid, pK_a 9.2
(C) Phenobarbituric acid, pK_a 7.9
(D) Salicylic acid, pK_a 3.0
(E) Sulfadiazine, pK_a 6.5

2. If 90.9 percent of a drug is in the nonionized form at pH 5, the pK_a of the drug is approximately

(A) 3
(B) 4
(C) 5
(D) 6
(E) 10

3. Drugs may be released slowly from various drug reservoirs over long periods of time. The body reservoir that holds the largest amount of the barbiturate thiopental is

(A) fat
(B) lung
(C) liver
(D) muscle
(E) serum albumin

4. Drug accumulation will occur after repeated injections if a drug is

(A) not metabolized by the liver
(B) administered intravenously
(C) administered at the $t_{1/2}$ of the drug
(D) distributed quickly into the extracellular space
(E) significantly protein-bound in the plasma

5. The route of excretion for drugs or their metabolic derivatives that is quantitatively the LEAST significant is which of the following?

(A) Biliary tract
(B) Kidneys
(C) Lungs
(D) Feces
(E) Milk

6. Oxidizable drugs form a complex with and are oxidized by which of the following iron-containing pigments in the microsomal fraction of liver?

(A) Cytochrome *a*
(B) Cytochrome *b*
(C) Cytochrome *c*
(D) Cytochrome c_1
(E) Cytochrome P-450

Questions 7-9

The following values were obtained for a patient:

24-hour urine volume	= 720 ml
concentration of creatinine in 24-hr urine specimen	= 0.6 mg/ml
concentration of creatinine in plasma	= 6.0 mg/100 ml

7. The patient's creatinine clearance (C_{Cr}) is

(A) 5 ml/min
(B) 10 ml/min
(C) 20 ml/min
(D) 60 ml/min
(E) 120 ml/min

8. A creatinine clearance value of 100 ml/min is a sign of which of the following conditions?

(A) Normal renal function
(B) Mild renal failure
(C) Severe renal failure
(D) Severe hepatic damage
(E) Mild cardiac toxicity

9. In the presence of impaired renal function, the time interval between maintenance doses needs to be lengthened for all the following antibiotics EXCEPT

(A) erythromycin
(B) streptomycin
(C) sulfisoxazole
(D) chlortetracycline
(E) ethambutol

Questions 10-13

Three hundred mg of a drug were administered intravenously to a 50-kg woman. The plasma concentration was then determined at intervals of time, as shown in the graph below.

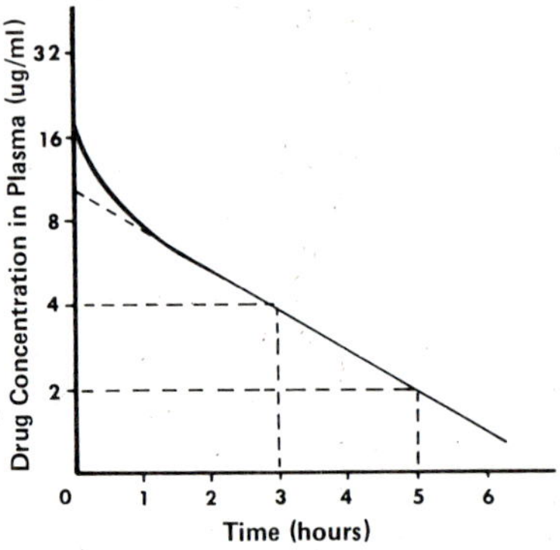

10. The apparent volume of distribution of the drug administered is

(A) 3 liters
(B) 10 liters
(C) 30 liters
(D) 50 liters
(E) 300 liters

11. The half-time ($t_{1/2}$) of clearance of the drug is

(A) 30 minutes
(B) 1 hour
(C) 2 hours
(D) 3 hours
(E) 4 hours

12. The elimination rate constant (k_e) of the drug is

(A) 0.1 hr^{-1}
(B) 0.2 hr^{-1}
(C) 0.35 hr^{-1}
(D) 0.69 hr^{-1}
(E) 1.38 hr^{-1}

13. The total body clearance of the drug is

(A) 0.2 liter/hr
(B) 0.5 liter/hr
(C) 1.0 liter/hr
(D) 3.0 liters/hr
(E) 10.5 liters/hr

14. If a drug has an elimination half-time ($t_{1/2}$) of 25 hr and 10 mg is administered intravenously every 12 hr, the expected average total body store of drug would be how many times greater than the 10 mg dose?

(A) 1.5
(B) 3.0
(C) 4.5
(D) 6.0
(E) 12.0

15. Assume that drug X is not significantly bound to plasma proteins and is excreted exclusively by the kidneys. If drug X is cleared from the body at a rate of 50 ml/min, which of the following conclusions is correct?

(A) Drug X is filtered by the glomeruli and reabsorbed in the tubules
(B) Drug X must be metabolized before excretion
(C) Renal blood flow should be increased
(D) The pH of urine must be alkaline
(E) None of the above

16. Phase 2 clinical studies of a drug are for the purpose of

(A) first administering it to humans
(B) establishing its efficacy and proper dosage schedules
(C) investigating its metabolic fate in humans
(D) conducting multi-institution trials with a large number of patients
(E) obtaining final FDA approval for marketing

17. Prescriptions for Schedule IV drugs, such as meprobamate (Miltown, Equanil), are subject to which of the following restrictions?

(A) They are not refillable
(B) They are refillable up to five times
(C) They are refillable without limit
(D) They can be dispensed only by hospital pharmacies
(E) They can be dispensed only by the Drug Enforcement Administration (DEA)

18. The transformation illustrated below is an example of which of the following detoxification mechanisms?

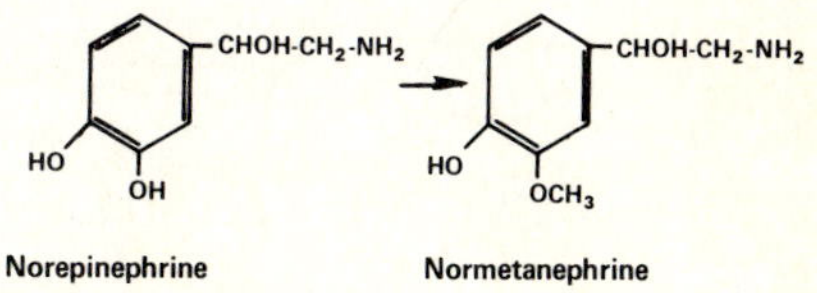

(A) Acetylation
(B) Esterification
(C) Hydrolysis
(D) Hydroxylation
(E) Methylation

19. The pharmacokinetic value that most reliably reflects the amount of drug reaching the target tissue after oral administration is

(A) peak blood concentration
(B) time to peak blood concentration
(C) product of the volume of distribution and the first-order rate constant
(D) volume of distribution
(E) area under the blood concentration-time curve

DIRECTIONS: Each question below contains four suggested answers of which **one** or **more** is correct. Choose the answer:

A	if	**1, 2, and 3**	are correct
B	if	**1 and 3**	are correct
C	if	**2 and 4**	are correct
D	if	**4**	is correct
E	if	**1, 2, 3, and 4**	are correct

20. From the graph below, which of the following statements are correct?

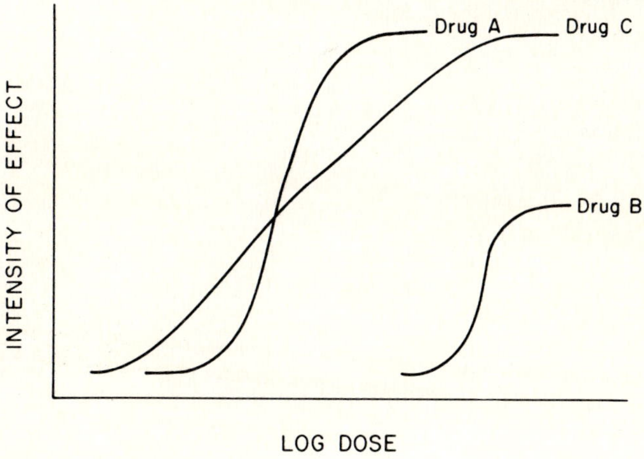

(1) Drug A is more potent than Drug B
(2) Drug A is less effective than Drug C
(3) Drug B is less effective than Drug C
(4) Drug A is more selective than Drug B

21. Agents that appear to act via cellular receptors include

(1) mannitol
(2) halothane (Fluothane)
(3) ethylenediaminetetraacetic acid (EDTA)
(4) cimetidine (Tagamet)

22. Monitoring the blood levels of a drug is particularly important if the

(1) interpatient variability is considerable
(2) therapeutic index of the drug is low
(3) biological effect is difficult to monitor
(4) drug has a short duration of action

SUMMARY OF DIRECTIONS

A	B	C	D	E
1, 2, 3 only	1, 3 only	2, 4 only	4 only	All are correct

23. Biotransformation reactions classed as nonsynthetic include which of the following?

(1) Oxidation
(2) Reduction
(3) Hydrolysis
(4) Acetylation

DIRECTIONS: The groups of questions below consist of lettered choices followed by several numbered items. For each numbered item select the **one** lettered choice with which it is **most** closely associated. Each lettered choice may be used once, more than once, or not at all.

Questions 24-26

For each description of a drug response that follows, choose the term with which it is most likely to be associated.

(A) Supersensitivity
(B) Tachyphylaxis
(C) Tolerance
(D) Hyposensitivity
(E) Anaphylaxis

24. Immunologically mediated drug reaction observed soon after drug administration

25. A rapid reduction in the effect of a given dose of a drug after only one or two doses

26. Hyperreactivity to a drug seen as a result of denervation

Questions 27-31

For each description that follows, select the transmembranal transport mechanism it best defines.

(A) Filtration
(B) Passive diffusion
(C) Facilitated diffusion
(D) Active transport
(E) Endocytosis

27. Lipid-soluble drugs cross the membrane at a rate proportional to the concentration gradient across the membrane and the lipid:water partition coefficient of the drug

28. Bulk flow of water through membrane pores, resulting from osmotic differences across the membrane, transports drug molecules that fit through the membrane pores

29. Drugs are transported by a membrane carrier that exhibits selectivity, competition, saturability. The movement is with the concentration gradient, and no energy is required

30. Cell membranes engulf droplets of solutions that are released inside the cell

31. By a selective saturable process requiring energy, molecules are transported across an electrochemical gradient

Questions 32-34

For each type of incompatibility described below; select the pair of substances that illustrates it.

(A) Tetracycline and milk
(B) Phenobarbital (Luminal) and secobarbital (Seconal)
(C) Isoproterenol (Isuprel) and propranolol (Inderal)
(D) Soap and benzalkonium chloride (Ionil)
(E) Doxycycline (Vibramycin) and chlortetracycline (Aureomycin)

32. Therapeutic incompatibility

33. Physical incompatibility

34. Chemical incompatibility

Questions 35-39

Many families of drugs consist of members that vary only with respect to substituents on a common ring structure. For each type of pharmacologic effect that follows, select the ring structure with which it is most likely to be associated.

A
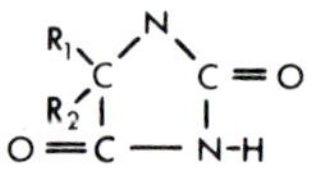

B
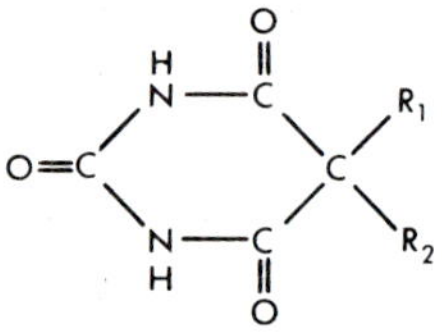

C
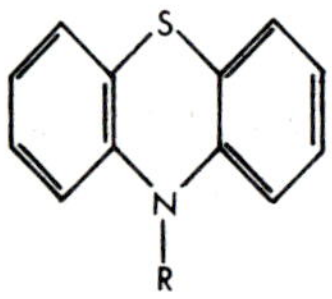

D
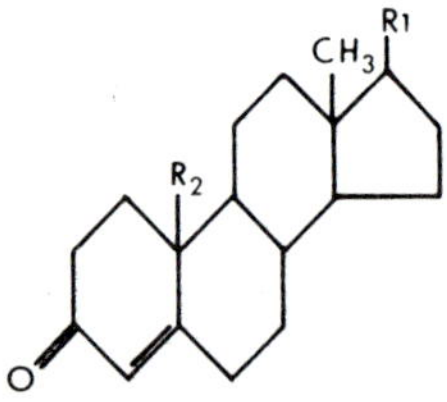

E
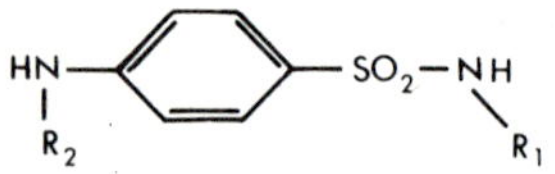

35. Antibiotic
36. Antipsychotic
37. Hypnotic
38. Oral contraceptive
39. Antiepileptic (petit mal)

Questions 40-44

For each description that follows, choose the drug with which it is most likely to be associated.

(A) Chloramphenicol
(B) Doxycycline
(C) Erythromycin
(D) Methenamine mandelate
(E) Penicillin G

40. This drug, which normally is excreted as glucuronide by the kidneys, reaches toxic levels in newborn infants deficient in glucuronyl transferase

41. This drug becomes concentrated in the liver and is excreted in an active form in the bile

42. Can inhibit hepatic microsomal enzymes and increase the half-times and toxicity of other drugs metabolized by this system

43. Usually prepared as a potassium salt, it may contribute to a potassium imbalance in the presence of renal failure

44. Although systemically nontoxic, this drug is contraindicated in the presence of moderate to severe renal failure because it potentiates uremic acidosis

General Principles Answers

1. The answer is B. *(Gilman, ed 6. p 4.)* The neutral nonionized form of a drug passes through a cellular membrane more easily than the ionized form because it is more lipid soluble. Thus, the rate of passive transport varies with the proportion of the drug that is nonionized. When the pH of a drug's environment is equal to its pK_a, the drug is half-dissociated. At an alkaline intestinal pH of about 8, of the drugs listed in the question, boric acid has the greatest percentage of its molecules in the nonionized form. The pH in the gastrointestinal tract is the major factor in absorption of many drugs. Weak acids (e.g., salicylates, barbiturates) are more readily absorbed from the stomach than from the other intestinal regions because these weak acids are mostly nonionized in the acidic environment of the stomach. The higher the value of the pK_a, the less ionized these acidic substances are in the stomach.

2. The answer is D. *(Goth, ed 10. pp 16-17.)* The Henderson-Hasselbalch equation defines the pK_a and can be expressed as

$$pK_a = pH + \log \frac{(\text{percent of drug not ionized})}{(\text{percent of drug ionized})}$$

$$pK_a = 5 + \log \frac{(90.9)}{(9.1)}$$

$$pK_a = 5 + 0.99952$$

$$pK_a = 5.99952$$

The transfer of drugs across membranes is dependent upon the pH of the internal environment and upon the pK_a of the drug. As the degree of ionization increases for an acidic drug, the smaller the value of the pK_a and the less the drug is permeable in membranes.

3. The answer is A. *(Gilman, ed 6. pp 9-10.)* Body fat may contain up to 70 percent of an administered dose of lipid-soluble thiopental three hours after injection. Other drugs may tend to accumulate in muscle or liver. For example, the concentration of the antimalarial drug quinacrine can be one thousand times greater in liver than in plasma. Serum albumin binds many drugs, some to appreciable degrees, thus reducing the free fraction that is pharmacologically effective. Plasma-bound drugs are readily released as the effective components are consumed by biotransformation or excretion. Drugs are usually released much more slowly from fat because fat has a relatively limited blood supply.

4. **The answer is C.** *(Gilman, ed 6. pp 21-23.)* The elimination of most drugs from the body can be described as a first-order process. Thus a constant fraction of the drug present at a given moment is removed per unit time. Almost 94 percent of a drug is eliminated by four half-times ($t_{1/2}$) and, consequently, administration of drug after this time does not result in significant drug accumulation. In contrast, if the drug is administered at intervals shorter than the time necessary for its complete elimination, the drug will accumulate in the body regardless of route of administration, distribution, or metabolic fate.

5. **The answer is E.** *(Gilman, ed 6. pp 20-21.)* The amounts of drugs excreted in milk are small compared to those excreted by other routes; but drugs in milk may have significant, undesired pharmacologic effects on breast-fed infants. The principal route of excretion of the products of a given drug varies with the drug. Some drugs are predominantly excreted by the kidneys, whereas others leave the body in the bile and feces. Inhalation anesthetic agents are eliminated by the lungs. The path of excretion may affect the clinical choice of a drug, as is the case with renal failure or hepatic insufficiency.

6. **The answer is E.** *(Gilman, ed 6. pp 13-16.)* The smooth-surfaced endoplasmic reticulum of liver cells contains enzymes that oxidize some drugs and is found in the microsomal fraction of liver homogenates. Microsomal enzymes contain glucuronide transferases, oxidases, and some reductases and hydrolases. Cytochrome P-450 complexes with the drug to be oxidized (usually a lipophilic drug) and, with molecular oxygen and reduced cytochrome *c* reductase, oxidizes numerous functional groups. Oxidative reactions include: *N*- and *O*-dealkylation; aliphatic and aromatic hydroxylation; *N*-oxidation and *N*-hydroxylation; sulfoxide formation; deamination; and desulfuration. Cytochrome P-450 was so named because it absorbs light at 450 nm when complexed to carbon monoxide.

7. **The answer is A.** *(Curry, ed 3. pp 210-212.)* Creatinine clearance (C_{Cr}) is expressed in units of ml/min and is calculated according to the formula

$$C_{Cr} = \frac{(U_{Cr})\,(V)}{P_{Cr}}$$

where U_{Cr} represents the urinary concentration of creatinine in units of mg/ml, V represents the urine flow rate in units of ml/min, and P_{Cr} represents the plasma concentration of creatinine in mg/ml. After converting, where necessary, the data given in the question into appropriate units, the values for the terms of the formula are: U_{Cr}, 0.6 mg/ml (normal: 0.67 to 1.7); V, 0.5 ml/min (normal:

0.42 to 0.83); and P_{Cr}, 0.06 mg/ml (normal: 0.6 to 1.2). After substitution of the values into the formula, the answer is calculated as follows:

$$C_{Cr} = \frac{(0.6 \text{ mg/ml})\ (0.5 \text{ ml/min})}{0.06 \text{ mg/ml}} = 5.0 \text{ ml/min.}$$

Normal values for creatinine clearance range from 87 to 139 ml/min.

8. **The answer is A.** *(Gilman, ed 6. p 1682.)* Creatinine clearance provides an accurate index of renal function. Normal values for a 70 kg man are 100-120 ml/min. The maintenance interval for the doses of drugs that are excreted by the kidneys must be lengthened according to the degree of renal failure.

9. **The answer is A.** *(Gilman, ed 6. p 1094.)* Because the majority of antibiotics are excreted by the kidney, in the presence of renal dysfunction it is imperative that the time interval between maintenance doses be prolonged in order to avert the accumulation of toxic blood levels of these agents. Erythromycin, which is metabolized by the liver, is exempt from this precaution. The four other antibiotics listed in the question, however, are excreted or inactivated primarily by the kidneys, and the time interval between maintenance doses must be prolonged when renal insufficiency occurs. This is especially important, inasmuch as many of these agents are toxic to the kidneys.

10. **The answer is C.** *(Gilman, ed 6. pp 21-23.)* In the example given in the question, a hypothetical plasma concentration of the drug at zero time of 10 μg/ml, or 0.01 mg/ml, can be estimated by the extrapolation of the linear portion of the elimination curve back to zero time. The apparent volume of distribution is that volume in which the drug would seem to be distributed if it existed in that volume at the same concentration as in the plasma. The apparent volume of distribution (V_d) is calculated by the following formula:

$$V_d = \frac{\text{Total amount of drug administered}}{\text{Concentration of drug in plasma}} = \frac{300 \text{ mg}}{0.01 \text{ mg/ml}} = 30 \text{ liters.}$$

In the example given, the drug is distributed throughout the entire body water.

11. **The answer is C.** *(Gilman, ed 6. pp 22-23.)* The half-time ($t_{1/2}$) of drug elimination in the example appearing in the question is two hours. At three hours after administration, the plasma concentration of the drug is 4 μg/ml; at five hours the concentration is 2 μg/ml. Thus, in two hours the plasma concentration of the drug decreased by one-half, and the half-time, or half-life, of the drug is two hours. The half-time is independent of the drug concentration and dosage. In addition, decay occurs according to first order kinetics: a linear relationship is obtained when the drug concentration is plotted on a **logarithmic** scale as a function of the time plotted on an **arithmetic** scale (a semilogarithmic plot).

12. The answer is C. *(Gilman, ed 6. pp 22-23.)* The fractional change in drug concentration per unit time is expressed by the elimination rate constant k_e. This constant is related to the half-time, designated as $t_{½}$, by the equation

$$k_e t_{½} = 0.693.$$

The units of the elimination rate constant are time $^{-1}$, while the $t_{½}$ is expressed in units of time. By substitution of the appropriate value for half-time derived from the graph into the above equation, rearranged to solve for k_e, the answer is calculated as follows:

$$k_e = \frac{0.693}{t_{½}} = \frac{0.693}{2\ \text{hr}} = 0.35\ \text{hr}^{-1}$$

13. The answer is E. *(Gilman, ed 6. pp 22-23.)* The total body clearance (C) is the product of the volume distribution of the drug (V_d) and the elimination rate constant (k_e). It is an expression of the volume of the V_d cleared per unit time. The more rapidly a drug is cleared, the greater is the value of C.

$$C = V_d k_e = (30\ \text{liters})(0.35\ \text{hr}^{-1}) = 10.5\ \text{liters/hr}$$

14. The answer is B. *(Gilman, ed 6. pp 23-24.)* With continuous or repeated drug administration, the total body store of drug increases in an exponential manner until a plateau is reached. The average total body store of drug at the plateau depends upon the dose (D), dosage interval (T), and the elimination half-time of the drug ($t_{½}$) and can be described by the following formula:

$$\text{average body store} = \frac{1.44\ (t_{½})\ D}{T} = \frac{1.44\ (25\ \text{hr})\ (10\ \text{mg})}{(12\ \text{hr})} = 30\ \text{mg}.$$

Thus, if a drug is administered at intervals equal to its elimination half-time, its concentration (average body store/volume of distribution) at the plateau phase will be 1.44 times that reached after a single dose.

15. The answer is A. *(Gilman, ed 6. pp 20, 885-887.)* In the average adult, the rate of glomerular filtration is approximately 125 ml/min. Free drugs that are eliminated by the kidneys at a lower rate (like the example in the question) must be undergoing tubular reabsorption.

16. The answer is B. *(Goth, ed 10. pp 46-47.)* Clinical trials that occur prior to marketing a drug have been loosely classified into 3 phases. Phase 1 studies involve relatively few human volunteers and investigators and are concerned with determining human toxicity, tolerated dosage range, drug metabolism, and distribution. The optimal treatment schedules and efficacy of the new drug are determined during Phase 2 studies performed by a larger number of clinical investigators. Large-scale clinical trials of the drug conducted in Phase 3 are designed to satisfy the FDA that the drug is safe and effective.

17. The answer is B. *(Goth, ed 10. p 751.)* The Federal Controlled Substances Act of 1970 provides that prescriptions for Schedule II drugs are not refillable, that Schedule III and IV drugs may be refilled up to five times within 6 months of initial issuance if authorized by the prescribing physician, and that Schedule V drugs may be refilled as often as the prescribing physician authorizes.

18. The answer is E. *(Goth, ed 10. pp 36-37.)* The detoxification example given in the question illustrates methylation of norepinephrine to inactive normetanephrine, which is excreted by the kidneys. The source of the methyl groups that are transferred to norepinephrine is *S*-adenosylmethionine, a sulfonium compound derived from ATP and methionine. Conjugation reactions, i.e., glucuronide or amino acid derivations, acetylation, and methylation, represent major paths for inactivating drugs and rendering them more susceptible to excretion by active enzymatic mechanisms that recognize the "added handle."

19. The answer is E. *(Gilman, ed 6. p 22. Goth, ed 10. p 22.)* The fraction of a drug dose absorbed after oral administration is affected by a wide variety of factors that can strongly influence the peak blood levels and the time to peak blood concentration. The volume of distribution and the total body clearance (volume of distribution x first-order elimination rate constant) also are important in determining the amount of drug that reaches the target tissue. Only the area under the blood concentration-time curve, however, reflects absorption, distribution, metabolism, and excretion factors and is the most reliable and popular method to evaluate bioavailability.

20. The answer is B (1, 3). *(Gilman, ed 6. pp 35-39.)* The log dose-effect curves for drugs allow comparisons of efficacy and potency. In the graph accompanying the question, the maximum biological effect of Drug A is equal to that of Drug C but more than that of Drug B. More of Drug B is required to produce a given effect compared to Drug A, and, thus, it is less potent than Drug A. No potency comparisons can be made between Drug A and C unless a dose or effect is mentioned, inasmuch as their slopes are not parallel. Selectivity of a drug refers to the relationship between the doses of a drug required to produce unwanted and desired effects; it can be measured as the margin of safety or therapeutic index of the drug. Neither can be determined from the above graph.

21. The answer is D (4). *(Gilman, ed 6. pp 35, 271, 277, 629-630, 1620-1621.)* Although many drugs exhibit a high affinity binding capacity to functional cellular components, some agents do not interact specifically with cellular receptors. For example, the primary mechanism of action of volatile general anesthetics, such as halothane, may be on the lipid matrix of biological membranes; mannitol acts by increasing the osmolarity of various body fluids; EDTA is effective as a detoxifying agent because it preferentially chelates metals, such as lead. Cimetidine, on the other hand, is a prototypic H_2-receptor blocking drug.

22. The answer is A (1, 2, 3). *(Gilman, ed 6. p 44.)* If a drug exhibits little interpatient variability in blood levels, results from previous pharmacokinetic studies can be used as a guide to dosage. Of those agents displaying considerable interpatient variability in absorption, distribution, metabolism, or excretion, most have sufficiently large therapeutic indices or marked therapeutic actions that careful monitoring of blood levels is not essential. Thus, with antibiotics like the penicillins, which have high therapeutic indices, the dose is increased to compensate for possible problems of interpatient variability; with analgesics, the dose is titrated to decrease pain.

23. The answer is A (1, 2, 3). *(Gilman, ed 6. p 12.)* Reactions involving the oxidation, reduction, or hydrolysis of a drug are classed as nonsynthetic. These reactions may result in either the activation or inactivation of a pharmacologic agent. Synthetic reactions, which almost always result in the inactivation of a drug, involve conjugation of the drug (or its active derivative) with an amino acid, carbohydrate, acetate, or sulfate. The conjugated forms of the drug or its derivative may be more easily excreted than the parent drug.

24-26. The answers are: 24-E, 25-B, 26-A. *(Goth, ed 10. pp 10, 49, 52-53, 122-123, 716-718.)* Anaphylaxis refers to an acute hypersensitivity reaction that appears to be mediated primarily by IgE. Specific antigens can interact with these antibodies and cause sensitized mast cells to release vasoactive substances, such as histamine. Anaphylaxis to pencillin is one of the best known examples; the drug of choice to relieve the symptoms is epinephrine.

Decreased sensitivity to a drug, or tolerance, is seen with some drugs such as opiates and usually requires repeated administration of the drug. Tachyphylaxis, in contrast, is tolerance that develops rapidly, often after a single injection of drug. In some cases this may be due to what is termed the down regulation of drug receptors, in which the number of receptors becomes decreased.

An individual who responds to an unusually low dose of a drug is called hyperreactive. Supersensitivity refers to increased responses to low doses only after denervation of an organ. At least three mechanisms are responsible for supersensitivity: increased receptors, reduction in tonic neuronal activity, and decreased neurotransmitter uptake mechanisms.

27-31. The answers are: 27-B, 28-A, 29-C, 30-E, 31-D. *(Gilman, ed 6. pp 3-5.)* The absorption, distribution, and elimination of drugs require that they cross various cellular membranes. The descriptions given in the question define the various transport mechanisms. The most common method by which ionic compounds of low molecular weight (100 to 200) enter cells is via membrane channels. The degree to which such filtration occurs varies from cell type to cell type because their pore sizes differ.

Passive diffusion is another mechanism by which substances cross membranes without the active participation of components in the membrane. Generally, lipid-soluble substances employ this method to enter cells. Both passive diffusion and filtration are dominant factors in most drug absorption, distribution, and elimination.

Carrier-mediated transport provides selectivity to the uptake process and is used to describe both active transport and facilitated diffusion. Active transport is responsible for the movement of a number of organic acids and bases across membranes of renal tubules, choroid plexuses, and hepatic cells. In contrast to active transport, facilitated diffusion does not require energy and so cannot prevail against a concentration gradient. Glucose transport into erythrocytes is a good example of this.

Pinocytosis is a type of endocytosis that is responsible for the transport of large molecules such as proteins and colloids. Some cell types—for example, endothelial cells—employ this transport mechanism extensively, but its importance in drug action is uncertain.

32-34. The answers are: 32-C, 33-D, 34-A. *(Gilman, ed 6. pp 188, 954, 978, 1187.)* Therapeutic incompatibility results when two drugs with opposing pharmacologic effects are administered. For example, a β-adrenergic stimulator will antagonize the effect of propranolol, a β-adrenergic blocking agent.

Physical incompatibility results when precipitation or another change in the physical state or solubility of a drug occurs. A common physical incompatibility takes place in the mixture of oppositely charged organic molecules, e.g., cationic and anionic detergents.

Chemical incompatibility results when two administered substances combine with each other chemically. Tetracyclines complex with calcium in milk, and with aluminum and magnesium which often are major components of antacids.

35-39. The answers are: 35-E, 36-C, 37-B, 38-D, 39-A. *(Goth, ed 10. pp 282, 335-336, 576, 583, 623.)* The five-membered hydantoin molecule is exhibited in Figure A (accompanying the questions), substitutions in the R_1 and R_2 positions providing the various derivatives, such as phenytoin (Dilantin), used in treating convulsive disorders. Trimethadione (Tridione), another derivative that, like phenytoin, is effective when administered orally, substitutes an oxygen atom for one nitrogen in the hydantoin ring, methylating the other.

Figure B illustrates the basic structure of barbituric acid, from which are derived the barbiturates, of which the first—barbital (Veronal)—was synthesized in 1903 by Emil Fischer and von Mering. The barbiturates are used both as hypnotics and anticonvulsants.

Figure C is the phenothiazine nucleus, attachments to the nitrogen atom of which account principally for the differences in the pharmacokinetics of the various phenothiazine derivatives. Examples include the piperazines, like prochlorperazine (Compazine), and the piperidines, like thioridazine (Mellaril).

Figure D shows the steroid polycyclic molecule that is the structural basis of androgens, estrogens, progestogens (synthetic progesterone derivatives, certain preparations of which are effective oral contraceptives), and some anti-inflammatory steroid agents.

Figure E illustrates sulfanilamide, the parent compound from which all the more therapeutically useful sulfonamides are derived. Some, like sulfadiazine, are short-acting ($t_{1/2}$ = 4 to 8 hours), others, like sulfamethoxazole, intermediate-acting ($t_{1/2}$ = 11 hours). Although among the earliest antibiotics to be developed, for certain disorders (e.g., acute infections of the urinary tract) the sulfonamides have retained their clinical importance.

Although it is not necessary to know the exact structure of each drug, knowledge of the basic structural characteristics of each class of drugs helps to categorize information and to predict the general properties and effects of some new preparations.

40-44. The answers are: 40-A, 41-C, 42-A, 43-E, 44-D. *(Gilman, ed 6. pp 1120, 1137, 1194-1195, 1223.)* Babies, especially premature ones, may lack glucuronyl transferase and therefore fail to conjugate chloramphenicol. Their kidneys cannot adequately excrete the unconjugated drug. Chloramphenicol can inhibit hepatic microsomal enzymes and reduce the metabolism of other drugs, such as phenytoin, dicumarol, and chlorpropamide. This has led to severe toxicity and, in some cases, death.

Erythromycin is concentrated by the liver and excreted in the bile. Very high concentrations of the active form of the antibiotic can be found in bile.

The potassium salt of penicillin G has 1.7 mEq K^+ per 1 million units. During a course of therapy, this amount of potassium constitutes a substantial load for a patient with severe renal failure.

Methenamine mandelate decomposes in the urine to formaldehyde and mandelic acid and helps to acidify the urine. In patients with renal failure, administration of this urinary tract antiseptic may lead to acidosis.

Chemotherapy

DIRECTIONS: Each question below contains five suggested answers. Choose the **one best** response to each question.

45. A 32-year-old man, who has smoked 2 packs of cigarettes a day for 10 years, presents with testicular carcinoma. His single breath diffusing capacity of carbon monoxide (DLco) is 50 percent below predicted values. Physical examination and chest x-rays suggest preexisting pulmonary disease. All the following drugs may be prescribed EXCEPT

(A) vinblastine (Velban)
(B) doxorubicin (Adriamycin)
(C) mithramycin (Mithracin)
(D) bleomycin (Blenoxane)
(E) *cis*-diamminedichloroplatinum (Platinol)

46. Kernicterus in newborn or premature infants treated with sulfonamides is due to

(A) enhanced synthesis of bilirubin
(B) displacement of bound bilirubin from albumin
(C) inhibition of bilirubin degradation
(D) inhibition of urinary excretion of bilirubin
(E) deposition of crystallin aggregates in the kidneys

47. Aluminum and calcium salts inhibit the intestinal absorption of which of the following agents?

(A) Isoniazid
(B) Chloramphenicol
(C) Phenoxymethyl penicillin
(D) Erythromycin
(E) Tetracycline

48. The preferred immunosuppressive drug for preventing the rejection of allografted kidneys is

(A) azathioprine
(B) cytosine arabinoside
(C) 5-fluorouracil
(D) 6-mercaptopurine
(E) vincristine

49. The drug most effective against malarial parasites in the liver (excluding erythrocytic phase) but not effective against parasites within erythrocytes is

(A) primaquine
(B) pyrimethamine
(C) quinacrine
(D) chloroquine
(E) chloroguanide

50. The release of formaldehyde is essential to the activity of which of the following drugs?

(A) Nalidixic acid
(B) Nifurtimox
(C) Nitrofurantoin
(D) Procarbazine
(E) Methenamine

51. Sulfisoxazole specifically inhibits which of the following processes?

(A) Conversion of tetrahydrofolic acid to dihydrofolic acid
(B) Conversion of deoxyuridine monophosphate to thymine ribonucleoside monophosphate
(C) Synthesis of methionine and serine
(D) Synthesis of pteroylglutamic acid
(E) Reduction of ribonucleotides

52. A 26-year-old man, complaining of severe headache, myalgia, and fever for the past four days, is admitted to the emergency room. Physical examination reveals an erythematous, macular rash that is most prominent over the wrists, ankles, palms, soles, and forearms. The patient reports that the onset of symptoms occurred soon after he had returned from a camping trip in western Virginia. The results of laboratory tests included: blood urea nitrogen, 55 mg/100 ml (normal: 10-20) and creatinine, 2.8 mg/100 ml (normal: <1.5). The initial diagnosis is Rocky Mountain spotted fever. The drug of choice is

(A) chloramphenicol
(B) tetracycline
(C) prednisone
(D) amphotericin B
(E) amantadine

53. The hemolytic anemia induced by large doses of penicillin is thought to be related to

(A) a direct toxic effect on the lipoprotein moiety of the red blood cell membrane
(B) poisoning of the red blood cell sodium-potassium pump
(C) circulating antipenicillin antibodies
(D) glucose 6-phosphate dehydrogenase deficiency
(E) denaturation of hemoglobin

54. Many patients who suffer hepatic failure and hepatic coma are treated with antibiotics, such as neomycin, that are not absorbed from the intestinal tract. The rationale for this treatment is that

(A) destruction of intestinal bacteria lessens the load of bacterial products, such as ammonia, that may be absorbed
(B) highly pathogenic bacteria, which often causes sepsis, are destroyed
(C) neomycin counteracts the hepatotoxic effect of absorbed bacterial by-products
(D) neomycin, in addition to acting as an antibiotic, acts as a diuretic agent by drawing third space fluid into the gut
(E) neomycin is indicated for ascending cholangitis, which is usually a factor in hepatic coma secondary to hepatic failure

55. In the diagram below, the site of action of penicillinase is

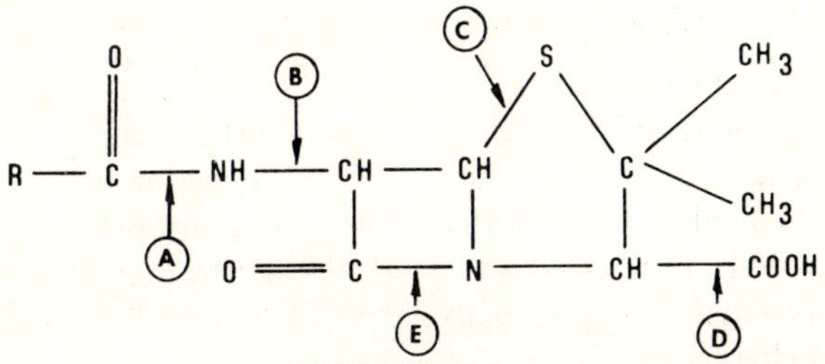

PENICILLIN G

(A) A
(B) B
(C) C
(D) D
(E) E

---

56. Clavulanic acid, a new type of β-lactam antibiotic, is important because it

(A) easily penetrates gram-negative microorganisms
(B) is specific for gram-positive micro-organisms
(C) is a potent inhibitor of cell wall transpeptidases
(D) inactivates bacterial β lactamases
(E) has a spectrum of activity similar to penicillin G

57. Pancytopenia is a common adverse reaction after administration of

(A) chloramphenicol
(B) chlorothiazide
(C) guanethidine
(D) methotrexate
(E) reserpine

58. A 24-year-old woman admitted to the emergency room complains of a severe, acute, generalized headache. She has a temperature of 40°C (104°F) and exhibits nuchal rigidity. Laboratory examination of her cerebrospinal fluid reveals gram-negative, kidney bean-shaped diplococci and 200 leukocytes/mm^3 (98 percent of which are polymorphonuclear neutrophils). The therapy of choice would be the administration of

(A) sulfonamides, intravenously
(B) amphotericin B, intravenously
(C) penicillin G, intravenously
(D) penicillin G, intrathecally
(E) chloramphenicol, intrathecally

59. Ethambutol is administered concurrently with streptomycin in the treatment of tuberculosis in order to

(A) reduce the pain of injection
(B) facilitate penetration of the blood-brain barrier
(C) retard the development of organisms resistant to streptomycin
(D) delay excretion of streptomycin by the kidney
(E) retard absorption after intramuscular injection

60. Antimetabolic drugs include all the following EXCEPT

(A) cyclophosphamide
(B) cytosine arabinoside
(C) 5-fluorouracil
(D) 6-mercaptopurine
(E) methotrexate

61. The tumor LEAST susceptible to "cycle-specific" anticancer agents is which of the following?

(A) Acute lymphoblastic leukemia
(B) Acute granulocytic leukemia
(C) Burkitt's lymphoma
(D) Adenocarcinoma of the colon
(E) Choriocarcinoma

62. The aminoglycoside most likely to remain a useful therapeutic agent in the event of streptomycin resistance is

(A) gentamycin
(B) amikacin
(C) neomycin
(D) tobramycin
(E) kanamycin

63. The drug used both in the treatment of active tuberculosis and most commonly in the chemoprophylaxis of tuberculosis is

(A) ethambutol
(B) cycloserine
(C) streptomycin
(D) isoniazid
(E) *p*-aminosalicylic acid

64. Which of the following statements about the neurotoxicity of the drug shown in the diagram below is true?

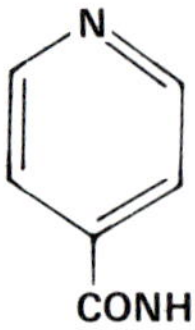

(A) It can be prevented by streptomycin
(B) It can be treated with vitamin B_{12}
(C) It is responsive to pyridoxine
(D) It manifests in the peripheral nervous system
(E) It occurs only in children

65. Candidiasis of the vagina, gastrointestinal tract, and oral cavity is treated primarily by which of the following drugs?

(A) Nystatin (Mycostatin)
(B) Miconazole (Monistat)
(C) Rifampin (Rifadin)
(D) Griseofulvin (Grisactin)
(E) Iodide

66. During the physical examination of a 32-year-old black man with chronic lymphocytic leukemia, the physician notes fluctuating levels of consciousness, nuchal rigidity, and an oral temperature of 38.3°C (101°F). Laboratory examination of the patient's cerebrospinal fluid discloses evidence of a cryptococcal infection, for which the patient receives appropriate doses of intravenous amphotericin B. Subsequently, a decreasing hematocrit develops that is best explained by which of the following statements?

(A) Chronic lymphocytic leukemia is frequently associated with anemia
(B) Fungal infection is frequently associated with anemia
(C) A common toxic reaction to amphotericin B is hemolytic anemia
(D) A common toxic reaction to amphotericin B is decreased erythrocyte production by bone marrow
(E) A common toxic reaction to amphotericin B is renal damage, which in turn depresses erythropoietin production

67. For treatment of a patient with typhus and impaired renal function, the agent of choice would be

(A) cephalothin
(B) minocycline
(C) clindamycin
(D) doxycycline
(E) penicillin G

68. A 23-year-old woman complains of persistent cough and fever. Physical examination reveals normal chest findings. She is found to have bullous myringitis and roentgenographic evidence of bilateral infiltration of the right lower lobe. Her physician diagnoses pneumococcal pneumonia and prescribes penicillin. In reviewing the case, another physician who knows that myringitis is seen with *Mycoplasma pneumoniae* infections would suggest alternative therapy with

(A) penicillin G
(B) tetracycline
(C) vancomycin
(D) gentamicin
(E) bacitracin

69. Cephalothin, one of several semisynthetic derivatives of cephalosporin C, has antibacterial activity based on a mechanism of action that includes

(A) interference with cross-linking of peptidoglycan strands
(B) competitive antagonism of pteroylglutamic acid synthesis
(C) functional alteration of 30 S ribosomal subunits
(D) inhibition of cephalosporinase activity
(E) inhibition of protein synthesis at the translation stage

70. Vertigo, inability to perceive termination of movement, and difficulty in sitting or standing without visual clues are some of the toxic reactions that are likely to occur in about 75 percent of patients who

(A) are allergic to penicillin
(B) receive tetracycline therapy
(C) receive amphotericin B therapy
(D) receive streptomycin therapy
(E) receive isoniazid therapy for tuberculosis

71. The nucleophilic attack on nitrogen 7 of guanine and the disruption of Watson-Crick base pairing patterns occur as a result of which of the following drugs?

(A) Cyclophosphamide
(B) Fluorouracil
(C) Methotrexate
(D) Prednisone
(E) Thioguanine

72. An anticancer agent that "takes advantage of" a qualitative difference between normal cells and some cancer cells is

(A) doxorubicin (Adriamycin)
(B) asparaginase
(C) cyclophosphamide (Cytoxan)
(D) fluorouracil
(E) methotrexate

73. Amantadine (Symmetrel), a synthetic antiviral agent used prophylactically against influenza A_2, is thought to act by

(A) preventing viral capsid protein production
(B) preventing virion release
(C) preventing penetration of the virus into the host cell
(D) preventing synthesis of nucleic acids
(E) causing lysis of infected host cells by release of intracellular lysosomal enzymes

74. Trypanosomiasis, or "sleeping sickness," can be successfully treated with arsenicals whose trypanocidal activity is thought to be due to

(A) interference with protein synthesis
(B) interference with glucose uptake
(C) interference with sulfhydryl-enzymes
(D) depletion of membrane lipoprotein precursors
(E) covalent binding of DNA

75. Griseofulvin is the agent of choice for treating

(A) *Candida* infections of the intestinal tract
(B) *Microsporum* infections of the hair
(C) *Actinomyces* infections of the cervicofacial region
(D) chromoblastomycosis caused by *Cladosporium*
(E) meningitis caused by *Coccidioides*

76. If phenoxymethyl and phenoxyethyl side chains are substituted on the 6-aminopenicillanic acid nucleus, penicillin V and phenethicillin are obtained, respectively. These penicillins have the same antibacterial spectrum as penicillin G. Their sole advantage over penicillin G is their

(A) decreased association with hypersensitivity reactions
(B) increased resistance to penicillinase
(C) increased resistance to penicillin amidase
(D) increased ability to enter the cerebrospinal fluid
(E) increased stability in acid solutions

77. Chloramphenicol is the drug of choice for the treatment of

(A) typhoid fever
(B) gonorrhea
(C) *S. aureus* infections
(D) anthrax
(E) gas gangrene

DIRECTIONS: Each question below contains four suggested answers of which **one** or **more** is correct. Choose the answer:

A	if	**1, 2, and 3**	are correct
B	if	**1 and 3**	are correct
C	if	**2 and 4**	are correct
D	if	**4**	is correct
E	if	**1, 2, 3, and 4**	are correct

78. Streptomycin and other aminoglycosides inhibit bacterial protein synthesis by binding to

(1) peptidoglycan units in the cell wall
(2) messenger RNA
(3) DNA
(4) 30 S ribosomal particles

79. Anthelmintic agents commonly interfere with parasitic

(1) motility
(2) division
(3) glycolysis
(4) membranes

80. Methisazone is a synthetic antiviral agent having properties that include

(1) activity against herpesvirus due to its capacity to inhibit both nucleoside reductase and DNA polymerase
(2) activity against poxvirus
(3) capacity to prevent the viral transmission of leukemia in mice
(4) usefulness in the treatment of eczema vaccinatum and vaccinia gangrenosa

81. The neurotoxicity of isoniazid is characterized by which of the following statements?

(1) It occurs in both slow and rapid acetylation
(2) It is enhanced by rifampin
(3) It can be reversed by pyridoxine
(4) It frequently produces convulsions in patients with no prior history of seizures

82. Accepted techniques for determining penicillin allergy include

(1) asking for a history of reactions
(2) skin testing with penicilloyl-polylysine
(3) skin testing with benzyl penicillin
(4) intravenous testing with minute quantities of penicillin G

83. An elderly, chronic alcoholic man in a comatose state was brought to the emergency room. The next day bilateral pulmonary infiltrates were noted on the x-ray film. Tracheal aspirate contained foul-smelling sputum and many gram-positive polymorphonuclear neutrophils and mixed flora. Appropriate antibiotic therapy in this case includes

(1) tetracycline
(2) penicillin G
(3) chloramphenicol
(4) cephalothin

84. Correct statements regarding chloramphenicol suppression of erythrocytic precursors include which of the following?

(1) Suppression is dose-related
(2) There is usually complete recovery after cessation of therapy
(3) The clinical picture is characterized by reticulocytopenia and a decrease in hemoglobin and plasma iron
(4) Marrow suppression is secondary to toxic suppression of erythropoietin production in the kidney

85. The design of combination chemotherapy protocols for anticancer agents frequently incorporates the principle that the drugs should

(1) be active against the tumor when used alone
(2) have different mechanisms of action
(3) have limited overlapping toxicities
(4) have different pharmacokinetic properties

86. Drugs used in the MOPP protocol for the treatment of Hodgkin's disease include

(1) prednisone
(2) vincristine
(3) procarbazine
(4) methotrexate

87. Penicillin has little or no antibacterial action against

(1) *Treponema pallidum*
(2) actively growing bacterial cells
(3) meningococci
(4) resting bacterial cells

88. Correct statements concerning asparaginase, an enzyme used in the chemotherapy of acute leukemia, include which of the following?

(1) It is derived from a mold
(2) It is capable of degrading a nonessential amino acid
(3) It is related to the antitumor antibiotics
(4) It is capable of influencing normal leukocytes

89. Antibiotics that are active in vitro against anaerobic bacteria such as *Bacteroides fragilis* include which of the following?

(1) Gentamicin (Garamycin)
(2) Lincomycin (Lincocin)
(3) Rifampin (Rifadin)
(4) Clindamycin (Cleocin)

90. Antibiotics that are primarily administered topically include

(1) neomycin
(2) polymyxin
(3) bacitracin
(4) streptomycin

91. Disseminated breast cancer that is estrogen-receptor positive has responded to antiestrogen therapy using

(1) diethylstilbestrol
(2) bleomycin
(3) fluoxymesterone
(4) tamoxifen

SUMMARY OF DIRECTIONS

A	B	C	D	E
1, 2, 3 only	1, 3 only	2, 4 only	4 only	All are correct

92. Correct statements about polymyxin B include which of the following?

(1) It is a surface-active agent
(2) It cannot be used topically
(3) It is active only against gram-negative bacteria
(4) It is an aminoglycoside antibiotic

93. The spread of resistance (R) plasmids by successive transfer from one microorganism to another is known to produce resistance to certain antibiotics. Antibiotics to which resistance develops by this method include

(1) tetracycline
(2) chloramphenicol
(3) erythromycin
(4) ampicillin

94. Cardiotoxicity limits the clinical usefulness of which of the following antitumor antibiotics?

(1) Dactinomycin (Cosmegen)
(2) Doxorubicin (Adriamycin)
(3) Bleomycin (Blenoxane)
(4) Daunorubicin (Cerubidine)

95. Methenamine mandelate (Mandelamine) acts as a urinary antiseptic by

(1) complementing the action of sulfonamides
(2) acidifying the urine
(3) releasing acetic acid
(4) liberating formaldehyde

96. Common complications of cephalothin therapy in hospitalized patients include

(1) fever, eosinophilia, and anaphylaxis
(2) hemolytic anemia characterized by a positive Coombs test result
(3) thrombophlebitis
(4) superinfection with gram-positive organisms

97. The acute toxic effects of methotrexate are reduced by the administration of

(1) ascorbic acid
(2) folic acid
(3) niacin
(4) folinic acid

98. True statements concerning the pharmacokinetics of allopurinol (Zyloprim) include which of the following?

(1) It can inhibit the metabolism of 6-mercaptopurine
(2) It can increase the antineoplastic action of 6-mercaptopurine
(3) It can inhibit xanthine oxidase
(4) It can act as a uricosuric agent

99. Correct statements about the clinical application of bacitracin include which of the following?

(1) It is rarely used parenterally and never orally
(2) It is bactericidal
(3) Topical application may aid in the treatment of infected dermal ulcers
(4) In contrast to vancomycin, it rarely causes significant nephrotoxicity

100. Resistance to penicillinase is found in which of the following penicillins?

(1) Ampicillin
(2) Oxacillin
(3) Carbenicillin
(4) Nafcillin

101. Stomatitis, a common complication of chemotherapy, may be expected after administration of

(1) methotrexate
(2) vincristine
(3) 5-fluorouracil
(4) bleomycin

102. Over 80 percent of patients who receive amphotericin B develop decreased renal function and abnormal urine sediments. This nephrotoxicity is associated with

(1) papillary necrosis
(2) renal vasoconstriction
(3) an immune complex glomerulonephritis
(4) a direct toxic effect on the tubules

103. Metronidazole is an effective treatment for which of the following infectious diseases?

(1) Amebiasis
(2) Pelvic inflammatory disease
(3) *Trichomonas* infections
(4) Moniliasis

104. Probenecid (Benemid) is sometimes given as an adjuvant in penicillin therapy because probenecid

(1) inhibits the renal tubular transport of penicillin
(2) has a synergistic bactericidal action with penicillin
(3) allows for higher serum levels of penicillin
(4) enhances the diffusion of penicillin through bacterial membranes

105. Thiabendazole (Mintezol), a benzimidazole derivative, is an anthelmintic drug used to treat infections caused by

(1) *Trichinella*
(2) *Trichuris*
(3) *Strongyloides*
(4) *Cestoda*

106. Causal prophylaxis of malarial infections may be achieved by treatment with

(1) 8-aminoquinolines
(2) acridine derivatives
(3) antifolics
(4) 4-aminoquinolines

107. Sulfonamides may cause renal damage that has been shown to be the result of precipitation of crystals in the collecting tubules of the kidney. Predisposing factors to such crystal formation include

(1) high urinary concentration of the drug
(2) low urinary solubility of the drug
(3) a urine pH of 5.0
(4) simultaneous administration of several sulfonamides

SUMMARY OF DIRECTIONS

A	B	C	D	E
1, 2, 3 only	1, 3 only	2, 4 only	4 only	All are correct

108. Pulmonary fibrosis may be associated with administration of which of the following chemotherapeutic agents?

(1) Bleomycin
(2) Hydroxyurea
(3) Busulfan
(4) Vincristine

109. Tetracyclines are the drugs of choice in the treatment of

(1) rickettsial disease
(2) mycoplasmal infection
(3) lymphogranuloma venereum
(4) gonorrhea

110. An infection caused by extraintestinal *Entamoeba histolytica* can be effectively treated with

(1) emetine
(2) paromomycin (Humatin)
(3) chloroquine
(4) glycobiarsol (Milibis)

111. Pharmacologic properties of amantadine (Symmetrel) include which of the following?

(1) It is a synthetic interferon
(2) It has a wide range of antiviral activity
(3) It is ineffective by oral administration
(4) It can prevent A_2 influenza virus infection

112. A 17-year-old girl develops watery diarrhea after a trip to Columbia. She is diagnosed as having amebic dysentery and treated with emetine hydrochloride. Correct statements concerning this therapy include which of the following?

(1) The drug is appropriate for the infection
(2) The drug causes marked symptomatic effects
(3) Treatment with the drug alone can convert the acute form of the disease to the chronic form
(4) The drug is particularly effective against enteric trophozoites

113. Advantages of deep intramuscular injection of benzathine penicillin G (Bicillin, Permapen) include which of the following?

(1) It can prevent group A streptococcal infection in patients with rheumatic heart disease
(2) It can prevent bacterial endocarditis after dental extraction in patients with known valvular disease
(3) It is useful in the treatment of syphilis
(4) It has a low incidence of allergic reactions when used in long-term therapy

114. Clinically established modes of penicillin resistance include

(1) penicillinase activity
(2) amidase activity
(3) permeability changes
(4) decarboxylase activity

115. The activity of dihydrofolate reductase obtained from protozoa or bacteria is inhibited by

(1) succinylsulfathiazole (Sulfasuxidine)
(2) trimethoprim
(3) sulfisoxazole (Gantrisin)
(4) pyrimethamine (Daraprim)

116. Respiratory paralysis is a life-threatening complication of neuromuscular blockade. The effect of neuromuscular blocking agents such as ether or tubocurarine is potentiated by which of the following antibiotics?

(1) Neomycin
(2) Polymyxin
(3) Streptomycin
(4) Penicillin

117. Bacterial protein synthesis is directly inhibited by which of the following antibiotics?

(1) Rifampin
(2) Chloramphenicol
(3) Penicillin
(4) Tetracycline

118. True statements concerning cephalosporin antibiotics include which of the following?

(1) Cephalosporins are bactericidal against multiplying bacteria
(2) Cephalosporins and penicillins have a similar spectrum of activity but no structural similarity
(3) Cross-hypersensitivity exists between cephalosporins and penicillins
(4) Unlike penicillins, cephalosporins are resistant to inactivation by β lactamase

119. Phenothiazine-induced agranulocytosis is characterized by

(1) a dose-related incidence
(2) an incidence of less than 1 in 10,000 patients
(3) onset within the first 90 days of therapy
(4) a higher incidence in women than men

120. The pharmacologic properties of amphotericin B include

(1) effectiveness when administered orally
(2) usefulness in the treatment of systemic mycoses
(3) binding to DNA
(4) severe renal toxicity

121. Drugs considered to be cell-cycle specific include

(1) 5-fluorouracil
(2) methotrexate
(3) 6-mercaptopurine
(4) vincristine

122. Antagonists of bacteriostasis induced by sulfonamides include

(1) acetylsalicylate
(2) folic acid
(3) pantothenic acid
(4) *p*-aminobenzoic acid

SUMMARY OF DIRECTIONS

A	B	C	D	E
1, 2, 3 only	1, 3 only	2, 4 only	4 only	All are correct

123. A serious toxic reaction of chloramphenicol known as the "gray syndrome" has occurred in newborn infants given large doses of the drug. Characteristics of this syndrome include which of the following?

(1) It is frequently fatal
(2) It is related to immature hepatic detoxification function
(3) It is related to inadequate renal excretory function
(4) It is characterized by life-threatening hyperthermia

DIRECTIONS: The groups of questions below consist of lettered choices followed by several numbered items. For each numbered item select the **one** lettered choice with which it is **most** closely associated. Each lettered choice may be used once, more than once, or not at all.

Questions 124-128

For each of the following drugs, select the characteristic with which it is most likely to be associated.

(A) A component of the MOPP regimen
(B) Orally administered alkylating agent
(C) Retained specifically in beta-cells of the islets of Langerhans
(D) Useful as a single agent against malignant melanoma
(E) An antitumor antibiotic that requires NADPH-dependent reduction

124. Streptozotocin
125. Dacarbazine (DTIC)
126. Mitomycin (Mutamycin)
127. Mechlorethamine
128. Lomustine (CCNU)

Questions 129-132

For each of the following antibiotics, select its appropriate mode of action.

(A) Binding to DNA-dependent RNA polymerase with inhibition
(B) Blocking transcription by binding to DNA
(C) Inhibition of binding of aminoacyl tRNA to 50 S ribosomal subunit
(D) Inhibition of peptide chain cross-linkage in bacterial cell walls
(E) Substitution for aminoacyl tRNA

129. Actinomycin
130. Chloramphenicol
131. Penicillin
132. Bacitracin

Questions 133-136

For each of the following chemotherapeutic agents, choose the neoplasm against which it is most likely to be effective.

(A) Chronic myelogenous leukemia
(B) Basal cell epithelioma
(C) Embryonal carcinoma
(D) Adrenal carcinoma
(E) Burkitt's lymphoma

133. Actinomycin D

134. Cyclophosphamide

135. Busulfan

136. Mitotane (Lysodren)

Questions 137-141

For each of the following drugs, select the adverse reaction with which it is most closely associated.

(A) Aseptic hemorrhagic cystitis
(B) Nephrotoxicity
(C) Myocardiopathy
(D) Peripheral neuropathy
(E) Pulmonary fibrosis

137. Doxorubicin (Adriamycin)

138. Bleomycin (Blenoxane)

139. Cyclophosphamide (Cytoxan)

140. *cis*-Diamminedichloroplatinum (Platinol)

141. Procarbazine (Matulane)

Questions 142-146

For each of the following parasites, select the drug that is most effective against it.

(A) Bithionol (Actamer)
(B) Piperazine (Antepar)
(C) Niridazole (Ambilhar)
(D) Diethylcarbamazine (Hetrazan)
(E) Niclosamide

142. *Enterobius vermicularis* (pinworms)

143. *Wuchereria bancrofti* (filariae)

144. *Paragonimus westermani* (lung flukes)

145. *Taenia saginata* (tapeworms)

146. *Schistosoma haematobium* (blood flukes)

Questions 147-151

Match the following.

(A) Oral drug of choice for penicillinase-producing bacteria
(B) Drug of choice for *Treponema pallidum*
(C) Broad-spectrum drug that is penicillinase sensitive
(D) Drug of choice for *Klebsiella pneumoniae*
(E) Permeability changes can cause resistance to this drug

147. Cephalothin

148. Penicillin G

149. Dicloxacillin

150. Carbenicillin

151. Methicillin

Questions 152-156

For each of the following drugs, select the toxicity with which it is most closely associated:

(A) Intermittent administration can result in jaundice or thrombocytopenia
(B) Pseudomembranous colitis
(C) Color blindness and blurred vision
(D) Nausea and vomiting
(E) Nephrotoxicity and vestibular effects

152. Clindamycin

153. Ethambutol

154. Rifampin

155. *p*-Aminosalicylic acid

156. Amikacin

Chemotherapy

Answers

45. The answer is D. *(Pratt, 1979. pp 184-185.)* The principal dose-limiting untoward effect of bleomycin is pulmonary toxicity. The mechanism of toxicity is uncertain. The clinical onset is characterized by decreasing pulmonary function, fine rales, cough, and diffuse basilar infiltrates, which may lead to severe, and sometimes fatal, pulmonary fibrosis. This complication develops in approximately 5 to 10 percent of individuals treated with bleomycin; about 1 percent of all patients receiving this drug die of pulmonary toxicity. Thus, extreme caution must be used in patients with a preexisting history of pulmonary disease. All the other drugs listed in the question are effective against testicular carcinomas and have not been associated with significant lung toxicity.

46. The answer is B. *(Gilman, ed 6. p 1114.)* Sulfonamides should not be used in neonates, especially premature infants, since the drug competes with bilirubin for serum albumin binding. This results in increased levels of free bilirubin causing kernicterus. Pregnant women at term also should not receive sulfonamides, owing to their ability to cross the placenta and enter the fetus in concentrations sufficient to produce toxic effects.

47. The answer is E. *(Gilman, ed 6. pp 1184-1185.)* Tetracyclines, as chelating agents, have a high affinity for the divalent cations of calcium and magnesium salts, for iron-containing preparations, for dairy products, and for aluminum hydroxide gels. The chelated complex is very insoluble and impairs absorption. Tetracyclines should be administered before meals to prevent formation of such chelates. Antacids that contain cations of calcium, magnesium, or aluminum should not be administered simultaneously with tetracyclines. These cations do not affect the absorption of the other drugs listed in the question.

48. The answer is A. *(Gilman, ed 6. pp 1251, 1286-1287.)* Azathioprine (Imuran), a derivative of mercaptopurine, is often used as an immunosuppressive drug; it is usually given in combination with prednisone to prevent renal allograft rejection. If toxicity or allergy to azathioprine develops in a patient who has had a renal transplant, cyclophosphamide is usually then given. The other agents listed in the question, including 6-mercaptopurine, generally are not used for immunosuppression.

49. The answer is A. *(Gilman, ed 6. p 1052.)* Primaquine is very active against exoerythrocytic forms of *P. vivax* and *P. falciparum*. While it exhibits some activity against asexual blood forms of *P. vivax*, results are variable. It is completely ineffective against asexual blood forms of *P. falciparum*. Primaquine is the agent of choice against late tissue forms of vivax malaria.

50. The answer is E. *(Gilman, ed 6. pp 1119-1120.)* Methenamine is a urinary antiseptic; it decomposes in acid medium to liberate formaldehyde. Its primary value is for treatment of chronic urinary tract infections that do not respond to such first-line drugs as sulfonamides or ampicillin. Nalidixic acid and nitrofurantoin are also used in chronic urinary tract infections, but these drugs have a different mechanism of action. Nifurtimox continues to be used as therapy for trypanosomiasis and is available from the Parasitic Disease Drug Service of the United States Center for Disease Control.

51. The answer is D. *(Gilman, ed 6. p 1108.)* Sulfonamides, as structural analogs of paraaminobenzoic acid, specifically inhibit the synthesis of folic acid (pteroylglutamic acid). This in turn leads to inhibition of protein, RNA, and DNA synthesis, and concomitant cessation of growth, because folic acid, in its cofactor form, is required for the synthesis of all these macromolecules. The fact that human cells do not contain folic acid synthetase is the basis for the selective toxicity of the sulfonamides.

52. The answer is A. *(Gilman, ed 6. p 1196.)* Both tetracycline and chloramphenicol are useful agents in the therapy of rickettsial infections. However, in the presence of renal insufficiency, the risk of injury to the liver by tetracyclines is greater than the risk of injury to the bone marrow by chloramphenicol. Therefore, for the patient described in the question, chloramphenicol is the drug of choice.

53. The answer is C. *(Gilman, ed 6. pp 1148-1149. Williams, ed 2. p 606.)* A hemolytic anemia occasionally occurs in patients receiving large doses of penicillin, often in the presence of renal failure. The anemia, characterized by a positive Coombs test result, is caused by the reaction of antipenicillin antibodies with penicillin bound to circulating red blood cells. Although an IgG antipenicillin antibody is usually responsible, other immunoglobulins (IgM, IgA) may be involved.

54. The answer is A. *(Gilman, ed 6. p 1178.)* In the prevention of hepatic coma, the mode of action of neomycin is best explained by its inhibition of ammonia production in the intestine. Oral administration of 4-8 g is acceptable provided renal function is normal. Owing to the possibility of severe renal insufficiency in the late stages of hepatic failure and of drug-induced ototoxicity, neomycin treatment should be carefully monitored.

55. The answer is E. *(Gilman, ed 6. p 1128.)* Penicillinase hydrolyzes the β-lactam ring of penicillin G to form inactive penicilloic acid. Consequently, the antibiotic is ineffective in the therapy of infections caused by penicillinase-producing microorganisms such as staphylococci, bacilli, *Escherichia coli, Pseudomonas aeruginosa,* and *Mycobacterium tuberculosis.*

56. The answer is D. *(Gilman, ed 6. p 1130.)* Clavulanic acid is a new antibiotic that is a potent inhibitor of β lactamases. The mode of inhibition is irreversible. Although clavulanic acid does not effectively inhibit the transpeptidase, it may be used in conjunction with a β-lactamase-sensitive penicillin to potentiate its activity.

57. The answer is D. *(Gilman, ed 6. pp 1193-1194, 1274.)* A major, predictable toxic reaction after administration of methotrexate is the suppression of bone marrow activity—manifested particularly by decreased granulocyte, platelet, and reticulocyte counts. Intensive methotrexate therapy requires monitoring of hematopoiesis and tests of renal and liver functions. Adverse effects of methotrexate can be reversed by the timely administration of folinic acid or leucovorin, the formyl derivative and active form of folic acid. The frequency of fatal pancytopenia in patients receiving chloramphenicol is very low (1:30,000). Nevertheless, great caution in the use of chloramphenicol is warranted because its effects are unpredictable and are not dose-related. Pancytopenia has been infrequently reported as an adverse effect following the administration of chlorothiazide, guanethidine, and reserpine.

58. The answer is C. *(Gilman, ed 6. pp 1135, 1139.)* The diagnosis after evaluation of the symptoms and signs described in the question is meningococcal meningitis. The therapy of choice is intravenous penicillin G, 20-24 million units per day for at least two weeks; intrathecal administration of penicillin G is no longer recommended. The majority of strains of *Neisseria meningitidis* are resistant to sulfonamides.

59. The answer is C. *(Gilman, ed 6. pp 1212-1214.)* An important problem in the chemotherapy of tuberculosis is bacterial drug resistance. For this reason, concurrent administration of two or more drugs should be employed to delay the development of drug resistance. Isoniazid (Nydrazid) is often combined with ethambutol (Myambutol) for this purpose. Streptomycin or rifampin (Rifadin) may also be added to the regimen to delay even further the development of drug resistance.

60. The answer is A. *(Gilman, ed 6. pp 1264-1266.)* Cyclophosphamide (Cytoxan) is a nitrogen mustard alkylating agent that typically reacts in electrophilic processes to form linkages with important biologic substances. Thus, cyclophosphamide damages DNA by causing miscoding, opening of the imidazole ring, and cross-linking of nucleic acid chains. Each of the other agents listed in the question is a metabolic inhibitor affecting the synthesis of DNA precursors. Cytosine arabinoside inhibits DNA polymerase. 5-Fluorouracil inhibits synthesis of deoxythymidine monophosphate (dTMP). 6-Mercaptopurine inhibits purine ring biosynthesis and nucleotide interconversions; methotrexate inhibits purine ring biosynthesis and dTMP synthesis.

61. The answer is D. *(Gilman, ed 6. p 1250.)* "Cycle-specific" cytotoxic agents are most effective in malignancies in which a large portion of the malignant cell population is undergoing mitosis. In leukemia, lymphoma, choriocarcinoma, and other rapidly growing tumors, these agents may induce a high percentage cell-kill of the entire tumor and at least of that portion of cells that are actively dividing. In slowly growing, solid tumors, such as carcinomas of the colon, the frequency of actively dividing cells is low, and perhaps the resting cells survive the cycle-specific agents and then can be recruited back into the proliferative cycle.

62. The answer is B. *(Gilman, ed 6. pp 1165, 1176.)* The most important mechanism of aminoglycoside resistance in bacteria is drug inactivation by microbial enzymes. Amikacin is uniquely resistant to these enzymes and, therefore, has the broadest spectrum of activity of all the aminoglycosides.

63. The answer is D. *(Gilman, ed 6. pp 1201, 1203.)* Isoniazid is the most effective tuberculostatic drug yet to be introduced. In controlled tests it has been shown to significantly decrease the incidence of clinical disease after known exposure to tuberculosis. Only actively growing bacilli are susceptible to the bactericidal property of isoniazid.

64. The answer is C. *(Gilman, ed 6. p 1202.)* The drug whose structure appears in the question is isoniazid, a commonly used antituberculous agent. Its most important side effects are related to peripheral and central nervous system toxicity. Peripheral neuritis occurs in 17 percent of patients receiving 6 mg/kg of isoniazid per day; the incidence is higher with larger doses. The effect is thought to be secondary to competition of the drug with pyridoxal phosphate for the enzyme apotryptophanase.

65. The answer is A. *(Gilman, ed 6. pp 1232-1233.)* Nystatin (Mycostatin) is used primarily to treat *Candida* infections of the skin, mucous membranes, and intestinal tract. The use of miconazole and iodide is restricted to topical application; griseofulvin is used primarily for skin mycoses. Nystatin is too toxic for parenteral use, but a closely related compound, amphotericin B, may be used systemically. Nystatin and amphotericin B interfere with membrane function in sensitive fungi by increasing its permeability to a number of small molecules.

66. **The answer is D.** *(Gilman, ed 6. pp 1235-1236.)* Amphotericin B can produce a normochromic, normocytic anemia characterized by decreased erythrocyte production. The blood picture usually becomes normal when treatment is discontinued. Very low concentrations of erythropoietin are associated with amphotericin-induced anemia. The occurrence of leukopenia or thrombopenia is quite rare.

67. **The answer is D.** *(Gilman, ed 6. p 1185.)* An agent of choice for rickettsial diseases is a tetracycline. Doxycycline is unique because, unlike other tetracyclines, it does not accumulate in patients with impaired renal function. It is excreted in the feces and is, therefore, one of the safest tetracyclines for treating extrarenal infections.

68. **The answer is B.** *(Gilman, ed 6. pp 1189-1190.)* Tetracycline is the drug of choice in the treatment of *Mycoplasma* infections. The antibiotics that act by inhibiting cell wall synthesis have no effect on *Mycoplasma* since the organism does not possess a cell wall. Tetracyclines are also effective in rickettsial and bacterial diseases and in infection produced by *Chlamydia.*

69. **The answer is A.** *(Gilman, ed 6. pp 1129, 1151.)* Cephalosporins, which include cephalothin, cefazolin, and cephalexin, appear to have a mechanism of action similar to that of the penicillins. Cephalosporins interfere with the final step (the transpeptidation reaction) in cell wall biosynthesis of susceptible bacteria. As a consequence of this type of interference, susceptible bacterial cells lose the rigidity of their cell walls that is provided by peptidoglycan and undergo lysis. Cephalosporins, because of their content of 7-aminocephalosporanic acid, are more stable in dilute acid solution than penicillins, and this characteristic leads to higher plasma levels after administration of equivalent doses. The cephalosporins are also more resistant to β lactamases compared to most penicillins.

70. **The answer is D.** *(Gilman, ed 6. p 1172.)* Streptomycin and other aminoglycosides can elicit toxic reactions involving both the vestibular and auditory branches of the eighth cranial nerve. Vestibular disturbance is detectable in nearly 75 percent of patients given 2 g of streptomycin daily for 2 to 4 months. Patients receiving an aminoglycoside should be monitored frequently for any hearing impairment owing to the irreversible deafness that may result from its prolonged use. None of the other agents listed in the question adversely affect the eighth cranial nerve function.

71. **The answer is A.** *(Gilman, ed 6. pp 1256, 1264.)* Cyclophosphamide (Cytoxan), an alkylating, nitrogen mustard type of bifunctional chemotherapeutic agent, reacts with purine and pyrimidine bases of DNA to form bridges and dimers. These products interfere with DNA replication. 5-Fluorouracil, metho-

trexate, and 6-thioguanine are antimetabolites, and the steroid prednisone has some tumor-suppressive effects. Cyclophosphamide is probably the most widely used alkylating agent.

72. The answer is B. *(Gilman, ed 6. p 1297.)* Although most normal tissues synthesize L-asparagine, in certain malignancies (such as acute lymphoblastic leukemia) this amino acid cannot be synthesized. Asparaginase, injected into patients who have such malignancies, acts to deprive the leukemic cells of this amino acid, and the malignant cells die whereas normal tissue is unaffected. The use of asparaginase, an enzyme that cleaves asparagine into aspartic acid and ammonia, was fortuitously discovered through injections of guinea pig serum (which contains the enzyme) into leukemic mice, whose tumors thereby were suppressed. Pharmacologic preparations of pure L-asparaginase are obtained from *Escherichia coli*. Allergic reactions occur in 5 to 20 percent of patients who were treated with this bacterial enzyme; in 5 to 50 percent of treated patients, toxic reactions affecting the kidneys, pancreas, the central nervous system, and the clotting mechanism have been reported.

73. The answer is C. *(Goth, ed 10. pp 656-657.)* Amantadine (Symmetrel) is thought to inhibit the penetration of infectious nucleic acid of influenza A virus strains into the host cell. In vitro, it is effective against influenza and rubella viruses. Amantadine both reduces the frequency of illness and diminishes the serologic response to influenza infection.

74. The answer is C. *(Gilman, ed 6. pp 1072-1074.)* Arsenicals, such as melarsoprol, are thought to interfere with the action of sulfhydryl-containing enzymes, specifically glucokinase. The trypanosomes can develop resistance to some organic arsenicals by decreasing the permeability of that particular drug. However, they usually remain sensitive to other arsenicals having different organic radicals. Melarsoprol, which, along with new nonarsenical trypanocides, has replaced the older arsenicals in much of the world, is particularly effective in treating the meningocephalic stage of trypanosomiasis owing to its penetration of the meninges.

75. The answer is B. *(Gilman, ed 6. pp 1237-1238.)* Griseofulvin is deposited in keratin precursor cells and persists tightly bound to keratin. As a result, the new growth of hair is resistant to fungal infection. *Microsporum, Trichophyton,* and *Epidermophyton* infections of the skin, hair, and nails are responsive to griseofulvin. The drug has no effect on other fungi, bacteria, yeasts, *Nocardia,* or *Actinomyces.*

76. The answer is E. *(Gilman, ed 6. pp 1131-1133.)* Compared to penicillin G, penicillin V and phenethicillin have increased stability in acid solutions. Consequently, there is greater and more reliable absorption from the gastrointestinal tract of these compounds than of penicillin G after oral administration. Penicillin V and phenethicillin are phenoxymethyl derivatives and phenoxyethyl analogs, or congeners, of penicillin G, respectively. They are available only for oral administration and thus do not replace parenteral penicillin.

77. The answer is A. *(Gilman, ed 6. pp 1191-1196.)* Chloramphenicol, an inhibitor of bacterial protein synthesis, is the agent of choice for the treatment of typhoid fever. Oral administration of 1 g every 6 hours for 4 weeks is indicated for adults. Recently, however, epidemics in some parts of the world due to *S. typhi* have resulted in a growing resistance of this organism to this drug.

78. The answer is D (4). *(Gilman, ed 6. pp 1164-1165.)* The bactericidal activity of streptomycin and other aminoglycosides involves a direct action on the 30 S ribosomal subunit, the site at which these agents both inhibit protein synthesis and diminish the accuracy of translation of the genetic code. Originally, misreading of the code was thought to be responsible for the lethal effects of aminoglycosides on bacteria. This concept has been discarded and the bactericidal effects of the aminoglycosides have yet to be explained.

79. The answer is B (1, 3). *(Pratt, 1977. pp 373-407.)* For most infections due to worms, the pathogenic forms of the parasite that are most susceptible to chemotherapy are the adult, nongrowing stages of the parasite's life cycle. Consequently, unlike all the antitumor agents and most antimicrobial agents, drugs that inhibit cell division are not generally effective anthelmintics. In contrast to the polymyxins (Aerosporin) and the polyene antibiotics, such as amphotericin B (Fungizone), anthelmintics do not act primarily on the cell membrane. The principal targets of the anthelmintics are either the mechanisms essential for the motor activity of the organism (motility) or the metabolic reactions that generate energy (glycolysis).

80. The answer is C (2, 4). *(Gilman, ed 6. p 1242.)* A synthetic antiviral agent, methisazone was reported in 1950 as active against poxviruses in chick embryos and mice and in 1960 as active against variola virus in mice. The clinical effectiveness of methisazone in the **prevention** of smallpox was first tested in a 1963 smallpox epidemic in India; the infectious disease developed in only 0.27 percent (3 of 1,100) of the persons who received the drug. Although of possible use in the treatment of vaccinia gangrenosa and eczema vaccinatum, methisazone has not proved useful in treating poxvirus infections. The drug is not available for use in the United States.

81. The answer is B (1, 3). *(Gilman, ed 6. p 1202.)* No conclusive evidence exists that the degree of isoniazid-induced neurotoxicity depends upon the rate of isoniazid acetylation in patients receiving the drug daily. The neurotoxicity of isoniazid resembles that of pyridoxine deficiency and is reversed by as little as 6 mg per day of the vitamin. Isoniazid increases the excretion of pyridoxine, thereby causing low plasma levels. Convulsions in patients with no previous history of seizures are rare.

82. The answer is A (1, 2, 3). *(Gilman, ed 6. p 1149.)* The most reliable criterion in determining penicillin allergy is a history of an allergic reaction to penicillin administration. Skin testing with both major and minor determinants has been useful in providing reasonable assurance against the occurrence of an immediate-type reaction. However, following intravenous test doses, a fatal reaction has been described with only 0.01 unit of penicillin. Penicillin has become the most common cause of anaphylactic shock.

83. The answer is A (1, 2, 3). *(Gilman, ed 6. pp 1139, 1151, 1183, 1195.)* As described in the question, the clinical setting and the character of the tracheal aspirate indicate aspiration pneumonia. By definition, pulmonary infection secondary to aspiration includes the presence of anaerobic organisms. Tetracycline, penicillin G, and chloramphenicol are active against most mouth flora and are sometimes used in combination clinically. Cephalothin is ineffective against anaerobes.

84. The answer is A (1, 2, 3). *(Gilman, ed 6. pp 1193-1194.)* The most common side effect of chloramphenicol therapy on the bone marrow is anemia, which occurs when blood levels of the drug are 25 μg/ml or higher. Recovery usually occurs approximately 12 days after the cessation of therapy. Chloramphenicol prevents the uptake of ^{59}Fe by normoblasts.

85. The answer is A (1, 2, 3). *(Pratt, 1979. pp 54-55.)* In general, combinations of anticancer agents are selected on the basis of the activity of each agent used alone, and a lack of similar host toxicities to the individual agents. In addition, it is believed that different mechanisms of action allow agents to act in a synergistic manner by operating on different sites or cell populations. Rarely have pharmacokinetic considerations been employed in designing new combination chemotherapeutic protocols.

86. The answer is A (1, 2, 3). *(Gilman, ed 6. pp 1289-1290.)* The drugs used in the MOPP regimen include mechlorethamine (Mustargen), vincristine (Oncovin), procarbazine (Matulane), and prednisone (Delta-Dome). Mechlorethamine is given intravenously and may cause nausea and vomiting. Vincristine is also given intravenously and is associated with adverse effects that include hair loss and neuromuscular disturbances. Procarbazine and prednisone are given orally. The administration of this combination of drugs in a defined cyclical schedule is the treatment of choice for stages III and IV of Hodgkin's disease and can be curative. The MOPP regimen is the standard against which other combination drug protocols for the treatment of Hodgkin's disease are measured.

87. The answer is D (4). *(Gilman, ed 6. pp 1129-1130.)* Because penicillins have no effect on existing bacterial cell walls, the bacteria must be multiplying in order for the bactericidal action of penicillin to occur. *Treponema pallidum* and meningococci are very susceptible to the action of penicillin G, the drug of choice for treating infections caused by these organisms. Bacteria such as *Mycobacterium tuberculosis* grow slowly and, even though they contain peptidoglycan, are not affected by penicillin G.

88. The answer is C (2, 4). *(Gilman, ed 6. p 1297.)* Asparaginase is an oncolytic enzyme that was initially purified from guinea pig serum but now is commercially purified from *E. coli.* Although most normal tissues synthesize sufficient quantities of L-asparagine, some malignant cells, in particular acute lymphoblastic leukemic cells, require exogenous amounts of this dibasic amino acid. Because asparaginase degrades L-asparagine, the malignant cells are deprived of this necessary amino acid and thus die. The use of asparaginase is limited, however, to acute lymphoblastic leukemia because of host toxicities that include anaphylaxis. L-Asparaginase also affects both T- and B-lymphocyte functions and has immunosuppressive activity.

89. The answer is C (2, 4). *(Gilman, ed 6. pp 1225-1226. Goth, ed 10. p 652.)* Lincomycin (Lincocin) and clindamycin (Cleocin) have demonstrated activity against *Bacteroides fragilis.* Neither gentamicin nor rifampin has demonstrated this activity. Clindamycin is often used when infection by anaerobic organisms is suspected and has superseded lincomycin as the drug of choice because it has greater activity with fewer side effects.

90. The answer is A (1, 2, 3). *(Gilman, ed 6. pp 1177, 1228, 1232.)* Neomycin, polymyxin, and bacitracin, in combination, are available as an over-the-counter ointment for the treatment of minor skin infections. Neomycin is too toxic for parenteral use; another aminoglycoside such as gentamicin is preferred. Polymyxin is occasionally administered parenterally for treatment of *Pseudomonas* infections. Because of its systemic toxicity, bacitracin is used almost exclusively in topical form.

91. The answer is D (4). *(Pratt, 1979. p 214.)* Tamoxifen is an antiestrogen that has been effective in treating postmenopausal women who have disseminated breast carcinomas that are estrogen-receptor positive. It can be administered orally, and its most common untoward effects include hot flashes, nausea, and vomiting. Diethylstilbestrol, a nonsteroidal estrogen, and fluoxymesterone, an androgen derivative, have also been used successfully to treat postmenopausal women with breast cancer.

92. The answer is B (1, 3). *(Gilman, ed 6. p 1228.)* In vitro and in vivo antibacterial activity of polymyxin B is restricted to gram-negative bacteria. Polymyxin B is a surface-active agent that produces a disorientation of bacterial lipoprotein membranes, so that they no longer function as effective osmotic barriers but allow the cell contents to leak out. Polymyxin B is most commonly used as a topical antibiotic because parenteral use produces severe side effects.

93. The answer is E (all). *(Gilman, ed 6. pp 1083-1084.)* Gram-positive and gram-negative bacteria can acquire drug resistance through resistance (R) plasmids. R factors provide different degrees of drug resistance from one host cell to another and from one R factor to another. Among the antibiotics to which resistance can develop by spread of R factors are sulfonamides, streptomycin, tetracyclines, chloramphenicol, kanamycin, neomycin, erythromycin, and ampicillin.

94. The answer is C (2, 4). *(Gilman, ed 6. pp 1291, 1293, 1295.)* Dactinomycin, effective in treating Wilms' tumor in children, is the oldest of the antitumor antibiotics listed in the question. It has mucosal and a variety of dermatologic side effects, as well as gastrointestinal and hematologic toxicity; bleomycin exhibits pulmonary toxicity and adverse effects on the oral mucosa. The anthracycline antibiotics, including daunorubicin and doxorubicin, share a propensity to cardiotoxicity that is dose related and exacerbated by irradiation. The risk of cardiotoxicity increases greatly with cumulative doses of doxorubicin greater than 550 mg/m^2 and with doses of daunorubicin greater than 750 mg/m^2. The cardiomyopathy may be due to lipid peroxidation in cardiac cells.

95. The answer is C (2, 4). *(Gilman, ed 6. pp 1119-1120.)* Methenamine mandelate (Mandelamine) is a compound salt of mandelic acid and methenamine, both of which are urinary antiseptics. Mandelic acid acts by acidifying the urine, and methenamine acts by slowly releasing formaldehyde in acidic solutions. Methenamine mandelate is useful for long-term suppressive treatment of urinary tract infections.

96. The answer is B (1, 3). *(Gilman, ed 6. pp 1156-1157.)* In about 5 percent of the patients receiving cephalothin, a hypersensitivity reaction develops that is characterized by fever, eosinophilia, serum sickness, rash, and anaphylaxis. A positive Coombs test result is also frequent but is seldom associated with hemolytic anemia. Thrombophlebitis with intravenous administration of cephalothin is almost universal. Pseudomonads and other gram-negative organisms that are resistant to cephalosporins are the most common cause of superinfections.

97. The answer is D (4). *(Gilman, ed 6. p 1273. Pratt, 1979. pp 103-105.)* The acute toxic effects of methotrexate can be reversed by the intramuscular administration of leucovorin calcium, or folinic acid, which is the active form and formyl derivative of folic acid. In some experimental therapeutic protocols for the treatment of central nervous system leukemia, very large doses of methotrexate will be administered that are capable of crossing the blood-brain barrier. In addition, large doses of methotrexate occasionally are used to maintain the remissions of patients who have acute lymphoblastic leukemia. In animal studies, the therapeutic index of methotrexate appears to be improved by the administration of folinic acid several hours after the high dose of methotrexate is given. Normal cells thus are preferentially "rescued" from the toxic effects of methotrexate.

98. The answer is E (all). *(Gilman, ed 6. p 1286.)* Allopurinol is a very effective inhibitor of the enzyme that metabolizes xanthine and hypoxanthine to form uric acid. This enzyme, xanthine oxidase, also is responsible for the oxidation of 6-mercaptopurine. Allopurinol, by blocking this reaction, increases the exposure time of tumor cells to 6-mercaptopurine. Unfortunately, no therapeutic gain is obtained because the host toxicity of 6-mercaptopurine is also increased.

99. The answer is A (1, 2, 3). *(Gilman, ed 6. p 1232.)* Bacitracin is not absorbed via the gastrointestinal tract and is rarely used parenterally because it can cause severe nephrotoxicity. Topically, its poor percutaneous absorption is of benefit. The mechanism of bactericidal activity appears to be interference with the function of bacterial cell membranes.

100. The answer is C (2, 4). *(Gilman, ed 6. p 1134.)* Oxacillin and nafcillin are resistant to penicillinase; ampicillin and carbenicillin are not. Ampicillin and carbenicillin are broad spectrum penicillins while oxacillin and nafcillin are generally specific for gram-positive microorganisms. Use of pencillinase-resistant penicillins should be reserved for infections caused by penicillinase-producing staphylococci.

101. The answer is B (1, 3). *(Pratt, 1979. pp 110-111, 131.)* Stomatitis is caused by a variety of antimetabolites including the folate antagonist methotrexate and the pyrimidine analog 5-fluorouracil. This inflammation is neither a usual consequence of the antitumor antibiotic bleomycin nor a side effect of the vinca alkaloids vincristine and vinblastine, whose toxicities are neurologic and hematologic.

102. The answer is C (2, 4). *(Gilman, ed 6. p 1235.)* The nephrotoxicity of amphotericin B is caused by renal vasoconstriction and a direct toxic effect of the drug on the renal tubules. Hypokalemia and hyposthenuria may precede the development of azotemia. A tubular defect in acid excretion superimposed upon an ischemic kidney appears to underlie both the hypokalemia and the nephrocalcinosis that are characteristic of amphotericin B nephropathy.

103. The answer is B (1, 3). *(Gilman, ed 6. pp 1063, 1087.)* Metronidazole (Flagyl) is directly trichomonacidal and is also active against intestinal and extraintestinal *Entamoeba histolytica* and *Giardia lamblia.* It has no demonstrated activity against *Candida albicans* or bacteria. Untoward effects, such as nausea, headache, dry mouth and metallic taste, are often encountered but rarely require interruption of treatment.

104. The answer is B (1, 3). *(Gilman, ed 6. p 1135.)* Probenecid (Benemid), by inhibiting the tubular secretion of penicillin, usually increases and prolongs blood levels of penicillin. Probenecid does not have any direct antibacterial activity. Another means of prolonging the serum levels of penicillin is the administration of a repository preparation of penicillin G, such as penicillin G procaine or penicillin G benzathine.

105. The answer is A (1, 2, 3). *(Goth, ed 10. pp 684-685.)* Thiabendazole (Mintezol) has been shown to be effective against *Trichinella* larvae in muscle, *Strongyloides*, cutaneous larva migrans, *Ascaris*, and *Trichuris*. Adverse effects occur in as many as one third of patients treated and consist of nausea, vertigo, headache, and weakness. Treatment usually involves oral administration of 25 mg/kg bid for several days.

106. The answer is B (1, 3). *(Gilman, ed 6. p 1039.)* In malaria, a causal prophylactic agent is one that prevents the onset of symptoms by killing the parasites before they enter the bloodstream. 8-Aminoquinolines (primaquine), and to a much lesser extent antifolics (pyrimethamine), are active against primary tissue schizonts or primary exoerythrocytic stages and thus prevent erythrocytic invasion. 4-Aminoquinolines act on erythrocytic forms. Acridine derivatives act rapidly against erythrocytic forms and are not significantly active against tissue or sexual forms.

107. The answer is A (1, 2, 3). *(Gilman, ed 6. p 1113.)* Precipitation of sulfonamide crystals may form concretions that injure the tubular epithelium or the epithelium of the pelvis of the kidney and obstruct the flow of urine. The concretions are more frequently observed if the solubility of the drug in the urine is low, the pH of the urine is low, or the concentration of the drug in the urine is high. Simultaneous administration of several sulfonamides, each at less than half its normal concentration, permits an adequate bacteriostatic blood concentration to be reached without the risk of renal damage.

108. The answer is B (1, 3). *(Gilman, ed 6. pp 1269, 1289, 1295, 1299.)* Hydroxyurea (Hydrea) causes adverse reactions to the hematopoietic system and occasionally causes gastrointestinal, dermatologic, and neurologic disturbances. Bleomycin (Blenoxane) and busulfan (Myleran) cause injury to the lung, resulting in fibrosis. Pulmonary fibrosis, the most serious side effect of bleomycin, may appear in as many as 10 percent of patients receiving this agent. Although bone marrow suppression leading to thrombocytopenia is the principal toxic manifestation of busulfan, pulmonary fibrosis is among a number of less frequently occurring side effects associated with this agent. Untoward effects of vincristine (Oncovin) are chiefly neurotoxic.

109. The answer is A (1, 2, 3). *(Gilman, ed 6. pp 1189-1191.)* Tetracyclines and chloramphenicol are therapeutically active in rickettsial infections. *Mycoplasma* and members of the lymphogranuloma-psittacosis group are also sensitive to tetracyclines. Although penicillin G is the drug of choice for gonorrhea, the presence of a dangerous degree of hypersensitivity to this agent is an indication for the administration of a tetracycline.

110. The answer is B (1, 3). *(Goth, ed 10. pp 678-681.)* Emetine and chloroquine are effective agents for the treatment of extraintestinal amebiasis and are, in general, ineffective for the treatment of intestinal infection. Paromomycin, an aminoglycoside antibiotic, and glycobiarsol are used to treat intestinal amebiasis and are ineffective in extraintestinal forms. Glycobiarsol, an arsenical, may evoke sensitivity to arsenic and is not currently available.

111. The answer is D (4). *(Gilman, ed 6. pp 1241, 1243.)* Amantadine (Symmetrel) is a synthetic crystalline amine of unusual structure. It is 90 percent absorbed after oral administration and has been shown to be clinically effective in the prevention of A_2 influenza virus infection. Interferons, on the other hand, are not virus specific; when induced by viral infection, they may suppress multiplication of a broad range of viruses.

112. The answer is A (1, 2, 3). *(Gilman, ed 6. p 1066. Goth, ed 10. pp 678-679.)* Emetine hydrochloride, a form of ipecac, is an emetic that is active against extraintestinal trophozoites and aids in controlling symptoms of acute amebiasis. It is not curative; upon termination of therapy, cysts can reappear in almost 50 percent of treated patients, who may become chronic, asymptomatic carriers. Cyst reappearance indicates that trophozoites still exist in the bowel. Emetine is a toxic drug that produces adverse reactions in cardiac and skeletal muscle. Its effects are cumulative, and it should not be administered for more than ten consecutive days.

113. The answer is B (1, 3). *(Gilman, ed 6. pp 1137-1139, 1141.)* The most effective agent for preventing the recurrence of rheumatic fever associated with group A β-hemolytic streptococcal infection (without bacteremia) is benzathine penicillin G (Bicillin, Permapen), administered by deep intramuscular injection only. The dosage may be either 1.2 million units once a month or 600,000 units every two weeks. For primary, secondary, and latent syphilis, the recommended dose is 2.4 million units by deep intramuscular injection. For upper respiratory streptococcal (group A) infections that may occur after dental procedures in patients who have valvular disease, the dose for adults is 1.2 million units and, for children over 60 pounds body weight, 900,000 units by deep intramuscular injection. Allergic reactions are at least as common and perhaps more common with benzathine penicillin G than with other penicillin derivatives.

114. The answer is B (1, 3). *(Gilman, ed 6. pp 1130, 1142.)* The primary mode of bacterial resistance to penicillin is by pencillinase production. Amidase activities, although they may exist, are minor and cannot protect the bacteria. Permeability changes in bacteria appear to be particularly important in the acquisition of resistance to methicillin.

115. The answer is C (2, 4). *(Gilman, ed 6. pp 1048-1049.)* The diaminopyrimidines trimethoprim and pyrimethamine are selective inhibitors of dihydrofolate reductase obtained from bacteria and protozoa. They have little effect on dihydrofolate reductase obtained from mammalian sources. The combination of a diaminopyrimidine and a sulfonamide is synergistic. The combination of trimethoprim and sulfamethoxazole is Bactrim, and its administration results in the inhibition of the activity of dihydrofolate reductase by trimethoprim and in the inhibition of bacterial synthesis of dihydrofolic acid by the competition between *p*-aminobenzoic acid and sulfamethoxazole.

116. The answer is A (1, 2, 3). *(Gilman, ed 6. pp 228-229, 1171, 1230.)* Colistin, lincomycin, and clindamycin—in addition to the first three antibiotic agents listed in the question—have been demonstrated to exert neuromuscular blocking effects that are synergistic with competitive blocking agents such as ether or tubocurarine. This effect is of clinical importance when these antibiotics are administered in large doses intravenously or intraperitoneally. Effects of overdosage include extended apnea and responses characteristic of histamine release.

117. The answer is C (2, 4). *(Gilman, ed 6. pp 1183, 1192. Goth, ed 10. p 619.)* Chloramphenicol and the tetracyclines inhibit protein synthesis by binding directly to the bacterial ribosome. Tetracyclines bind specifically to the 30 S subunit, whereas chloramphenicol binds to the 50 S subunit. Penicillin interferes with cell wall synthesis and rifampin inhibits DNA-dependent RNA polymerase.

118. The answer is B (1, 3). *(Gilman, ed 6. pp 1151, 1156.)* Both cephalosporins and penicillins contain a β-lactam ring, and both drugs are sensitive to inactivation by β lactamase to varying degrees. The mechanism of action of the two antibiotics is similar: cross-linking of D-alanyl-D-alanine of the peptidoglycan in the formation of bacterial cell walls is inhibited. Cross-allergenicity presumably occurs on the basis of hypersensitivity to similar breakdown products.

119. The answer is E (all). *(Craig, p 510.)* Phenothiazine-induced agranulocytosis occurs in less than 1 of 10,000 patients treated. It is dose-related and tends to occur in older women whose white blood cell counts were low before therapy was begun. If agranulocytosis is to appear, even during prolonged therapy, it occurs within the first 90 days. Marrow function recovers promptly after cessation of therapy.

120. The answer is C (2, 4). *(Gilman, ed 6. pp 1233-1236.)* Amphotericin B is poorly absorbed from the gastrointestinal tract. The agent's antifungal activity is contingent upon binding of the drug to a sterol moiety present in the membranes of sensitive fungi, thus changing their permeability. Over 80 percent of patients given amphotericin B develop decreased renal function and abnormal urine sediments. The side effects can be so serious that amphotericin B is restricted to the treatment of severe systemic fungal infections.

121. The answer is E (all). *(Gilman, ed 6. pp 1250, 1255. Pratt, 1979. pp 29-36.)* Cell-cycle specific drugs inhibit growth at some phase in the growth cycle. These phases are classified as follows: G_1, a presynthetic phase; S, the DNA synthesis phase; G_2, the interval following the end of DNA synthesis; M, the mitosis phase during which the G_2 cell divides into two G_1 daughter cells. Purine synthesis is inhibited by 6-mercaptopurine and by methotrexate; deoxythymidine monophosphate synthesis is blocked by 5-fluorouracil. Each of these three drugs affects the S phase of cell growth. Vincristine, however, blocks the cell cycle at the mitotic phase.

122. The answer is C (2, 4). *(Gilman, ed 6. p 1108.)* The mechanism of action of sulfonamides is thought to be through competitive antagonism of *p*-aminobenzoic acid, the utilization of which by bacteria is essential to folic acid synthesis. An excess of folic or *p*-aminobenzoic acid will overcome the bacteriostatic effect of sulfonamides. Bacteria that do not need folic acid or can use preformed folic acid are not affected by sulfonamides.

123. The answer is A (1, 2, 3). *(Gilman, ed 6. p 1194.)* The often fatal "gray syndrome" of chloramphenicol toxicity consists of abdominal distension, vasomotor collapse, diarrhea, rapid, irregular respirations progressing to flaccidity, ashen-gray color (due to pallid cyanosis), and hypothermia. It is related to the failure of chloramphenicol to be conjugated with glucuronic acid. Neonates have insufficient glucuronyl transferase for conjugation and inadequately developed renal mechanisms for effective excretion of the unconjugated drug.

124-128. The answers are: 124-C, 125-D, 126-E, 127-A, 128-B. *(Pratt, 1979. pp 78-79, 85, 88-89, 91, 174-178.)* Streptozotocin is a nitrosourea-like antibiotic that contains a glucosamine moiety that allows it to be selectively taken up by the β cells of the islets of Langerhans. Consequently, it appears to be useful in treating metastatic islet cell carcinoma. Insulin shock has been reported as a serious acute toxicity in some patients receiving streptozotocin.

Dacarbazine (DTIC) is a relatively new member of the triazene class of alkylating agents, which appear to require demethylation for activity. It has displayed significant antineoplastic action against malignant melanomas.

Mitomycin is a potent antibiotic that selectively inhibits DNA synthesis due to its ability to alkylate and cross-link DNA. Mitomycin has no effect on purified DNA in vivo; the addition of microsomes, however, activates mitomycin by an NADPH-dependent reduction of the quinone moiety on the drug. The reduced antibiotic undergoes spontaneous rearrangement and can form covalent bonds with nucleophilic groups in DNA, RNA, and proteins.

Mechlorethamine, the first widely used anticancer agent, has been largely susperseded by less toxic drugs. Nevertheless, this alkylating agent has an important role in the treatment of Hodgkin's lymphoma as a component in the chemotherapeutic regiment MOPP (mechlorethamine, vincristine (Oncovin), procarbazine, and prednisone).

Lomustine (CCNU) is a nitrosourea that is rapidly absorbed from the gastrointestinal tract and, thus, is orally active. From animal studies it appears that the plasma half-life of this compound is quite short (<6 minutes). Because of their lipophilicity, the nitrosoureas, including CCNU, cross the blood-brain barrier and have been used to treat malignancies of the central nervous system.

129-132. The answers are: 129-B, 130-C, 131-D, 132-D. *(Goth, ed 10. pp 619-620.)* In general, antibiotics work by interfering with cell wall, protein, or nucleic acid synthesis. Actinomycin D forms a complex with DNA, which involves selective binding at the cytosine-guanine segment, thus blocking DNA-dependent RNA synthesis.

Chloramphenicol, tetracycline, erythromycin, and the aminoglycosides inhibit protein synthesis through their effects on ribosomes. In the case of chloramphenicol, the binding of aminoacyl tRNAs to the ribosome is inhibited in bacteria. In mammalian cells, however, chloramphenicol only prevents the attachment of new mRNAs to the ribosome.

Penicillins as well as cephalosporins block the final step in the assembly of the mucopeptide of bacterial cell walls. Cycloserine affects cell wall synthesis through nucleotide intermediates (phase 1) and bacitracin through disaccharide intermediates (phase 2). Inhibition of cell wall synthesis results in lysis of the cell.

133-136. The answers are: 133-C, 134-E, 135-A, 136-D. *(Pratt, 1979. pp 154-155.)* Actinomycin D is an antitumor antibiotic that has been used against germ cell tumors for many years. It is given to patients who have localized disease (pathologic stage A) at the time of initial surgery and in prophylactic courses every two to three months postoperatively. This therapy is directed against the metastatic disease which, although inapparent at initial presentation, eventually occurs in 10 to 15 percent of patients and leads to death.

Cyclophosphamide, as a single agent, has been used for more than a decade against Burkitt's lymphoma, the childhood lymphoma that is seen chiefly in Africa. In either single large doses, or in lower weekly doses, this drug has produced tumor remission in more than 90 percent of affected patients. Cyclophosphamide must be activated by the mixed-function oxidase system of the smooth endoplasmic reticulum of the liver. Sterile hemorrhagic cystitis, a serious but reversible syndrome, occurs in 5 to 10 percent of patients treated with this agent.

Busulfan is an alkylating agent that has a time-honored role in the therapy of chronic myelogenous leukemia; it has been efficacious in prolonging and improving the quality of life in patients who have this disease. Busulfan is supplanted by hydroxyurea, dibromomannitol, and other agents used against acute myelogenous leukemia in the presence of refractory disease or blast crises.

Mitotane (Lysodren) has the chemical formula, 1,1-dichloro-2(*o*-chlorophenyl)-2(*p*-chlorophenyl)-ethane and the trivial name *o,p′*-DDD. Used to decrease the secretion of steroids by the adrenal cortex and against tumors derived from this tissue, mitotane has gastrointestinal, cutaneous, hepatic, and bone marrow toxicity. Nevertheless, it is still used against metastatic adrenal carcinoma with hypersecretion and produces tumor regression and significant palliation in approximately 35 percent of affected patients.

137-141. The answers are: 137-C, 138-E, 139-A, 140-B, 141-D. *(Gilman, ed 6. pp 1266, 1276, 1292-1294, 1298-1299. Pratt, 1979. p 249.)* Myocardiopathy with severe and progressive congestive heart failure occurs in over 20 percent of patients who receive a total dose of more than 550 mg/m^2 doxorubicin (Adriamycin). The congestive heart failure produced by doxorubicin is unresponsive to digitalis.

Pulmonary fibrosis occurs in 5 to 10 percent of patients who have received bleomycin (Blenoxane). The risk for cumulative doses below 400 units is not dose-related, but the risk increases rapidly for cumulative doses above 400 units in patients older than 70 years of age, and in patients who have preexisting pulmonary disease.

Aseptic hemorrhagic cystitis has been reported as an adverse reaction occurring in 5 to 10 percent of patients who receive cyclophosphamide (Cytoxan). This syndrome is usually reversible upon withdrawal of the drug; occurrence of this complication can be minimized by adequate fluid intake and frequent voiding.

The two major toxicities associated with *cis*-diamminedichloroplatinum, (Platinol), a drug used in treating testicular tumors, are vomiting and nephrotoxicity. The focal acute necrosis observed in the kidney affects primarily the distal tubules and collecting ducts. Mannitol or the high-ceiling diuretics are highly effective in opposing the renal toxicity induced by Platinol.

Procarbazine commonly produces a dose-related, reversible bone marrow depression including thrombocytopenia and leukopenia. Neurotoxicity is also associated with this drug in 10 to 20 percent of the patients receiving it. This is manifested as ataxia, disorders in consciousness, and peripheral neuropathies. Procarbazine can reduce plasma pyridoxal phosphate levels, a phenomenon that may be responsible for the neurotoxicity.

142-146. The answers are: 142-B, 143-D, 144-A, 145-E, 146-C. *(Gilman, ed 6. pp 1015, 1023, 1033-1035.)* Pinworm infestation should be treated with a piperazine compound in conjunction with rigid standards of personal hygiene. Piperazine is also the drug of choice against *Ascaris lumbricoides*.

Filariasis is effectively treated with diethylcarbamazine, a piperazine derivative, which both suppresses and, in most cases, cures the infection. The drug is inactive against *W. bancrofti* in vitro. However, in vivo activity appears to be due to a sensitization of the microfilariae toward phagocytosis by the fixed macrophages of the reticuloendothelial system.

Niclosamide is the agent of choice for treatment of *T. saginata* infections. It is highly effective and relatively free from side effects. These properties have resulted in its replacement of quinacrine, which has become obsolete.

Schistosomiasis responds well to antimony-containing compounds. However, *Schistosoma haematobium* is also sensitive to niridazole, a relatively new compound that is both schistosomicidal and amebicidal.

Bithionol has been found useful in the treatment of the lung flukes *P. westermani* and *P. kellicotti*. Treatment usually involves the oral administration of 40 to 50 mg/kg, in divided doses on alternate days, for a total of 10 to 15 doses. Chloroquine in large doses has also been successful in the therapy of lung flukes.

147-151. The answers are: 147-D, 148-B, 149-A, 150-C, 151-E. *(Gilman, ed 6. pp 1126-1157.)* Cephalothin is the cephalosporin most resistant to degradation by penicillinases. It is usually administered only intravenously because of pain following intramuscular injection and its poor absorption when given orally. Many investigators believe that cephalosporins are the only drugs of choice for *K. pneumoniae*.

Penicillin G, the least expensive of all the penicillins, is highly effective against gram-positive cocci but is readily hydrolyzed by penicillinase. It is the agent of choice in the treatment of syphilis (*T. pallidum*).

Dicloxacillin is a semisynthetic penicillin that is relatively stable in acidic media and is adequately absorbed after oral administration. It is also highly resistant to inactivation by penicillinase. Dicloxacillin is manufactured for oral use in capsules and as a suspension.

Carbenicillin is a penicillinase-sensitive β-lactam antibiotic. Its chief advantages are its relatively broad spectrum and its effectiveness against infections caused by *Pseudomonas, Proteus,* and other gram-negative microorganisms.

Methicillin is effective against nearly all strains of *S. aureus* by virtue of its resistance to pencillinase. Its acid-sensitivity makes oral administration relatively ineffective. There has been an increasing incidence of methicillin-resistant strains. Although the precise mechanism of resistance is not known, it appears to be related to decreased permeability of the cell wall to the antibiotic.

152-156. The answers are: 152-B, 153-C, 154-A, 155-D, 156-E. *(Gilman, ed 6. pp 1176, 1204-1205, 1207, 1210, 1226-1227.)* Clindamycin is similar to erythromycin in its in vitro activity against *Streptococcus pyogenes, Streptococcus viridans,* and pneumococci. A number of patients treated with clindamycin have developed pseudomembranous colitis, which is characterized by abdominal pain, fever, diarrhea, and mucus and blood in the stools. This syndrome is apparently due to the production of an exotoxin by clindamycin-resistant strains of *Clostridium difficile.*

Ethambutol, in combination with isoniazid, is useful in the therapy of tuberculosis. Although its mechanism of action is unknown, the most important side effect of ethambutol is optic neuritis, which causes a decrease in visual acuity and the loss of the ability to perceive the color green. The incidence of this effect is dose-dependent and recovery usually occurs upon withdrawal of the drug.

Rifampin inhibits the growth of most gram-positive and many gram-negative bacteria. Although untoward effects occur infrequently by routine administration, adverse effects have been associated with intermittent administration. These include a flu-like syndrome, thrombocytopenia, and jaundice that may be lethal.

p-Aminosalicylic acid is bacteriostatic and highly specific for *M. tuber-*

culosis, with a mechanism of action that appears to be very similar to that of the sulfonamides in other bacteria. The incidence of untoward effects with *p*-aminosalicylic acid is approximately 10 percent; these problems are predominantly gastrointestinal, including anorexia, nausea, epigastric pain, abdominal stress, and diarrhea.

Amikacin, the newest aminoglycoside antibiotic, is uniquely resistant to inactivating enzymes and has the broadest spectrum of all members of this class. However, like other aminoglycosides, amikacin has the potential to produce vestibular, cochlear, and renal toxicity.

Toxicology

DIRECTIONS: Each question below contains five suggested answers. Choose the **one best** response to each question.

157. In a patient who is not comatose, emesis is indicated after acute poisoning following oral ingestion of all the following EXCEPT

(A) strong acid or alkali
(B) antihistamines
(C) digitalis
(D) morphine
(E) diazepam (Valium)

158. The appearance of a Parkinson-like syndrome as a late effect is most likely to be associated with chronic inhalation of

(A) magnesium salt
(B) manganese salt
(C) calcium salt
(D) nickel salt
(E) lithium salt

159. Convulsions due to drug poisoning are most commonly associated with

(A) phenobarbital
(B) diazepam
(C) strychnine
(D) chlorpromazine
(E) phenytoin

DIRECTIONS: Each question below contains four suggested answers of which **one or more** is correct. Choose the answer:

A	if	**1, 2, and 3**	are correct
B	if	**1 and 3**	are correct
C	if	**2 and 4**	are correct
D	if	**4**	is correct
E	if	**1, 2, 3, and 4**	are correct

160. An ideal therapeutic chelating agent for the treatment of heavy metal poisoning should have which of the following properties?

(1) Solubility in water
(2) Capability of being readily excreted as a chelate
(3) Resistance to metabolic degradation
(4) Retention of chelating capacity at body fluid pH

161. Severe accidental poisoning by an organophosphate insecticide, such as parathion, should be treated with

(1) dimercaptopropanol (BAL)
(2) pralidoxime (2-PAM)
(3) ethylenediaminetetraacetic acid (EDTA)
(4) atropine

162. True statements about hydrocyanic acid (prussic acid) include which of the following?

(1) At low concentrations, it stimulates respiration
(2) It is converted in the body to thiocyanate
(3) Poisoning by it can be treated with sodium nitrite
(4) Poisoning by it can be treated with sodium thiosulfate

163. Activated charcoal may be used to treat poisoning due to

(1) primaquine
(2) aspirin
(3) propoxyphene
(4) sulfuric acid

164. Hemodialysis is highly effective in the treatment of severe poisoning with

(1) acetylsalicylic acid
(2) digoxin
(3) phenobarbital
(4) methaqualone (Quaalude)

165. True statements about persons who are suffering from carbon monoxide poisoning include which of the following?

(1) The oxygen-carrying capacity of blood is decreased
(2) The oxyhemoglobin dissociation curve becomes "shifted to the left"
(3) A carboxyhemoglobin blood level of less than 30 percent produces minimal symptoms
(4) Treatment with 100% oxygen is effective

SUMMARY OF DIRECTIONS

A	B	C	D	E
1, 2, 3 only	1, 3 only	2, 4 only	4 only	All are correct

166. Toxic side effects of chronic phenytoin (Dilantin) administration include

(1) nystagmus
(2) gingival hyperplasia
(3) osteomalacia
(4) megaloblastic anemia

167. Increased intracranial pressure may occur under which of the following conditions of drug therapy?

(1) Excessive chronic intake of vitamin A
(2) Excessive acute intake of sodium salicylate
(3) Usual therapeutic doses of tetracycline
(4) Very large doses of glycerin

168. The various salts of ethylenediaminetetraacetic acid (EDTA) can be used for which of the following purposes?

(1) Diagnosis of lead poisoning
(2) Diagnosis of mercury poisoning
(3) Treatment of lead poisoning
(4) Treatment of mercury poisoning

169. Ototoxicity may be associated with which of the following drugs?

(1) Ethacrynic acid
(2) Gentamicin
(3) Furosemide
(4) Streptomycin

170. Individuals who are deficient in glucose 6-phosphate dehydrogenase experience hemolysis following treatment with which of the following antibiotics?

(1) Chloramphenicol
(2) Nitrofurantoin
(3) Primaquine
(4) Sulfanilamide

171. Anesthetic agents that are contraindicated in patients who have acute intermittent porphyria include

(1) cyclopropane
(2) diethyl ether
(3) ketamine
(4) thiopental sodium

172. Side effects of oral contraceptives include

(1) impaired glucose tolerance
(2) increased blood pressure
(3) melasma
(4) induction of breast carcinomas

173. Direct hepatic toxicity has been observed with

(1) halothane (Fluothane)
(2) thiopental sodium (Pentothal)
(3) enflurane (Ethrane)
(4) nitrous oxide

DIRECTIONS: The groups of questions below consist of lettered choices followed by several numbered items. For each numbered item select the **one** lettered choice with which it is **most** closely associated. Each lettered choice may be used once, more than once, or not at all.

Questions 174-177

For each agent listed below, select the classification that is most appropriate.

(A) Procarcinogen
(B) Primary carcinogens
(C) Promoter
(D) Cocarcinogen
(E) Anticarcinogen

174. Ethanol

175. Nitrogen mustard

176. Benzo[a]pyrene

177. Bile salts

Questions 178-182

For each of the following agents, select its specific antidote.

(A) Leucovorin
(B) Naloxone (Narcan)
(C) Physostigmine
(D) Ethanol
(E) Diazepam (Valium)

178. Atropine

179. Strychnine

180. Methotrexate

181. Morphine

182. Ethylene glycol

Toxicology Answers

157. The answer is A. *(Doull, ed 2. pp 681-691. Gilman, ed 6. p 1609.)* Poisoning by oral ingestion of most substances usually should be treated by the rapid induction of emesis. It is contraindicated when the patient is comatose or convulsing, since the individual may aspirate gastric contents. If an emetic is employed after ingestion of strong acids or bases, additional necrosis of the esophagus and possible gastric perforation can occur. In some cases emesis is contraindicated after the ingestion of a CNS stimulant because further stimulation associated with vomiting may lead to convulsions.

158. The answer is B. *(Doull, ed 2. pp 200, 449-450.)* The acute toxicity associated with inhalation of manganese salts, usually in the form of manganese dioxide, is pneumonitis. Chronic inhalation, however, involves the central nervous system and produces a syndrome that closely resembles the extrapyramidal symptoms of parkinsonism. Chronic manganese poisoning can be treated with levodopa (Dopar).

159. The answer is C. *(Gilman, ed 6. p 587.)* Strychnine acts as a competitive antagonist of glycine, the predominant postsynaptic inhibitory transmitter in the brain and spinal cord. The fatal adult dose is 30 to 100 mg. Persons poisoned by strychnine suffer convulsions that progress to full tetanic convulsions in hyperextension. Because the diaphragm and thoracic muscles are fully contracted, the patient cannot breathe. Hypoxia eventually causes medullary paralysis and death. Control of the convulsions and respiratory support are the immediate objectives of therapy. Diazepam may be preferred to a barbiturate in controlling the convulsions because it offers less concomitant respiratory depression. Poisoning due to the other drugs listed in the question is not associated with convulsions but with central nervous system depression.

160. The answer is E (all). *(Gilman, ed 6. pp 1615-1616.)* All the properties listed in the question should be found in the ideal therapeutic agent for the treatment of heavy metal poisoning. In addition, such an agent should be able to penetrate to metal storage sites, form metal complexes that are less toxic than the free metal ion, and have a greater affinity for the metal ion than do endogenous ligands. Because in vivo systems are very complicated, the true evaluation of a chelating agent must be determined in clinical situations.

161. The answer is C (2, 4). *(Doull, ed 2. pp 374-375.)* The organophosphate insecticides inactivate acetylcholinesterase, which results in accumulation of endogenous acetylcholine in nerve tissue and effector organs. Very severe cases of acute poisoning should be treated first with atropine followed by intravenous pralidoxime (2-PAM). Atropine inhibits the actions of acetylcholine, whereas 2-PAM reactivates the inactivated acetylcholinesterase. The effectiveness of 2-PAM in reversing acetylcholinesterase inhibition in vivo depends upon early treatments inasmuch as the "aged" inhibited enzyme cannot be reactivated.

162. The answer is E (all). *(Gilman, ed 6. pp 1651-1652.)* At low concentrations, hydrocyanic acid (HCN, or prussic acid) inhibits the oxidative functions of chemoreceptors in the carotid and aortic bodies and stimulates respiration, much as do low P_{O_2} levels. Cyanide can produce cytotoxic hypoxia. Cyanide is eliminated chiefly in the form of thiocyanate ion, but this pathway is limited by the endogenous supply of thiosulfate. In cyanide poisoning, the administration of sodium nitrite forms methemoglobin ($Hb\text{-}Fe^{+++}$) that competes with cytochrome oxidase for the cyanide ion. After sodium nitrate infusion, sodium thiosulfate should be infused slowly over a period of ten minutes.

163. The answer is A (1, 2, 3). *(Gilman, ed 6. pp 954, 1610.)* Activated charcoal, a fine, black powder with a high adsorptive capacity, is considered to be a highly valuable agent in the treatment of many kinds of drug poisoning. Drugs that are well adsorbed by activated charcoal include primaquine, propoxyphene, dextroamphetamine, chlorpheniramine, and aspirin. Mineral acids, alkalies, tolbutamide, and other drugs that are insoluble in acidic aqueous solution are not well adsorbed.

164. The answer is B (1, 3). *(Doull, ed 2. pp 679-680. Gilman, ed 6. pp 359-360, 367, 696, 755.)* Hemodialysis is effective in treating cases of severe poisoning with barbiturates and salicylates. The long-acting barbiturates, which are less protein-bound than the short-acting ones, respond more effectively to hemodialysis. Hemodialysis significantly shortens the half-life of drug clearance and, consequently, the duration of coma. Together with hemoperfusion, exchange transfusion, and peritoneal dialysis, hemodialysis is useful in the treatment of salicylate poisoning. Drugs with large volumes of distribution or extensively bound to plasma proteins, such as digitalis or methaqualone, are not well removed by dialysis.

165. The answer is E (all). *(Gilman, ed 6. pp 1641-1643.)* Carboxyhemoglobin (COHb) causes a shift to the left in the dissociation curve of oxyhemoglobin (O_2Hb), releasing less oxygen to the tissues. A much lower tissue P_{O_2} becomes required for the dissociation of oxygen under this condition. When the COHb is less than 40 percent of blood hemoglobin, compensation at low oxygen tensions can occur. If COHb exceeds 40 percent of blood hemoglobin, the tissues cannot be adequately oxygenated. The preferred treatment for CO poisoning is the administration of 100 percent oxygen because the half-life of blood levels of COHb varies inversely with the P_{O_2}. Thus, oxygen administration results in an increased rate of dissociation of COHb.

166. The answer is E (all). *(Gilman, ed 6. p 454.)* Phenytoin (Dilantin) therapy is associated with many toxic side effects including nystagmus, gingival hyperplasia, osteomalacia, and megaloblastic anemia. The megaloblastic anemia results from the interference of phenytoin with folate absorption and metabolism. Osteomalacia seems to be a result of interference with vitamin D metabolism. Gingival hyperplasia results from altered collagen metabolism and is the most common toxic manifestation in children. Nystagmus, along with diplopia, vertigo, and ataxia are among the CNS symptoms attributable to toxic levels of phenytoin.

167. The answer is B (1, 3). *(Gilman, ed 6. pp 695-696, 1188, 1587.)* Signs of hypervitaminosis A may include increased intracranial pressure, an adverse effect that also may occur in young children who are receiving usual therapeutic dosages of tetracycline. The increased intracranial pressure due to tetracycline administration is manifested by a bulging of the fontanelles in young infants; this adverse reaction is reversed by ending the tetracycline therapy. The most prominent aspects of acute toxicity from sodium salicylate are disturbances in acid-base balance and electrolyte content in the plasma; increased intracranial pressure has not been reported. Very large doses of glycerin can result in hemolysis, hemoglobinuria, and renal failure.

168. The answer is B (1, 3). *(Gilman, ed 6. pp 1620-1628. Isselbacher, ed 9. pp 967-968.)* Calcium disodium ethylenediaminetetraacetic acid ($CaNa_2$ EDTA) is useful in both the diagnosis and the treatment of lead poisoning. By chelating lead and increasing its excretion in urine, $CaNa_2$EDTA both rids the body of lead and provides a method of measuring the lead burden in the body. $CaNa_2$-EDTA is relatively ineffective, however, in the treatment of mercury poisoning, despite the in vitro ability of mercury to displace calcium from $CaNa_2$EDTA. The concentrations of mercury in the plasma and urine provide a relatively good index of the total body burden of inorganic mercury. In addition, the sulfhydryl groups that are plentiful in hair bind and concentrate mercury, leaving a good record of mercury exposure.

169. The answer is E (all). *(Gilman, ed 6. pp 906, 1169-1174.)* Ototoxicity is associated with each of the drugs listed in the question. The administration of aminoglycoside antibiotics (such as gentamicin and streptomycin) in conjunction with high-ceiling diuretics (such as ethacrynic acid and furosemide) should be avoided not only because these diuretics can be ototoxic but also because they increase the ototoxicity of aminoglycoside antibiotics by increasing their levels in serum and tissue. Some cases of tinnitus and of reversible and irreversible hearing damage have occurred after furosemide was administered parenterally, then orally. Deafness and tinnitus have been reported as adverse effects of ethacrynic acid therapy, most frequently in patients who had severely impaired renal function and who had received high parenteral doses. Streptomycin therapy may cause nausea, vomiting, and vertigo at levels of intensity directly related to the dose and duration of treatment. Streptomycin is especially ototoxic in patients who are elderly and who have renal dysfunction.

170. The answer is E (all). *(Gilman, ed 6. p 1053. Isselbacher, ed 9. pp 1544-1545.)* More than 15 drugs have been associated with hemolysis in individuals who are deficient in glucose 6-phosphate dehydrogenase. The mechanism of hemolysis, although not fully understood, is thought to be related to drug-induced free radicals that denature hemoglobin and lead to oxidation of intrachain disulfide bridges. Hemoglobin is precipitated, and red blood cells are destroyed. With adequate glucose 6-phosphate dehydrogenase, oxidation is prevented by maintaining sufficient levels of nicotinamide adenine dinucleotide phosphate (reduced form) and (consequently) reduced glutathione. The defect is an example of genetically determined, individual variations in response to certain drugs.

171. The answer is D (4). *(Gilman, ed 6. p 294.)* Induction of anesthesia by parenteral administration of thiopental sodium (Pentothal) and other barbiturates is absolutely contraindicated in patients who have acute intermittent porphyria. In these patients, barbiturate administration exacerbates the symptoms due to the gastrointestinal and neurologic disturbances, causes extensive demyelination of peripheral nerves, and can lead to death.

172. The answer is A (1, 2, 3). *(Gilman, ed 6. p 1443. Goth, ed 10. pp 583-584.)* Adverse effects of oral contraceptives include: nausea and vomiting; elevation of blood pressure; skin reactions such as melasma, chloasma, and rash; disturbances in liver function and glucose tolerance; headache; and cerebral and visual disturbances. Mood depression has also been noted to occur. Thromboembolic disorders have been associated with oral contraceptives containing estrogen; these drugs interact with coumarin drugs, necessitating an increase in the normal therapeutic dosage of anticoagulants. Although evidence of estrogen induced vaginal and uterine carcinomas has been reported, most investigators have found no association between the usage of oral contraceptives and breast carcinomas.

173. The answer is B (1, 3). *(Gilman, ed 6. pp 282-291.)* Halothane and enflurane are effective general anesthetics; however, along with other halogenated compounds such as chloroform and carbon tetrachloride, they share a propensity to cause hepatotoxicity. Hepatic function is impaired during treatment with halothane and enflurane, but this is rapidly reversible upon termination of treatment. Hepatic necrosis may result from biotransformation of halothane and enflurane to reactive intermediates that react with liver macromolecules.

174-177. The answers are: 174-D, 175-B, 176-A, 177-C. *(Doull, ed 2. pp 86-114.)* Agents that participate in the induction of tumors can be classified mechanistically. Electrophilic substances, which directly interact with DNA, are called direct-acting or primary carcinogens. These included nitrogen mustard-like anticancer agents, epoxides, and some halogen-containing compounds.

Procarcinogens require metabolic activation to form the reactive electrophile. The polycyclic aromatic hydrocarbons, such as benzo [a] pyrene, must be "activated" by a cytochrome P-450 enzyme system called aryl hydrocarbon hydroxylase. This enzyme system can be readily induced by the polycyclic aromatic hydrocarbons.

Cocarcinogens, such as ethanol, are agents that must be administered together with primary carcinogens or a procarcinogen to increase the carcinogenic process. A cocarcinogen can increase nonspecifically the proliferation of cells that have been damaged by the primary carcinogen or they may alter the metabolism of the procarcinogen.

In contrast to cocarcinogen, substances like bile salts that can increase the carcinogenic process when administered after the primary carcinogen or the procarcinogen are called promoters. Promoters do not influence the process if administered prior to exposure to the carcinogen. Although some cocarcinogens are promoters, not all promoters are cocarcinogens.

178-182. The answers are: 178-C, 179-E, 180-A, 181-B, 182-D. *(Gilman, ed 6. pp 127-128, 510, 587, 1273, 1275, 1646-1647.)* The peripheral and central nervous system effects of atropine poisoning may be reversed with physostigmine. Because physostigmine is metabolized more rapidly than atropine, repeated doses may be necessary. Neostigmine and other quaternary anticholinesterase drugs that do not cross the blood-brain barrier cannot be used to treat the central nervous system effects of atropine.

In the event of strychnine toxicity, rapid therapy can prevent convulsions and support respiration. The convulsions can be controlled with intravenous diazepam and, if respiration remains inadequate, mechanical assistance may be required.

Methotrexate inhibits dihydrofolate reductase and limits the supply of N^5-formyltetrahydrofolate, which is required in the synthesis of thymine. Leucovorin (citrovorum factor or N^5-formyltetrahydrofolate) can protect against the toxic effects of methotrexate. Methotrexate therapy followed by leucovorin is a chemotherapeutic regimen for some neoplastic disorders.

Acute morphine poisoning is characterized by coma, pupils of pinpoint size, and depressed respiration. Intravenous injection of the opiate antagonist, naloxone, is the treatment of choice since it has no direct respiratory depressant effects. Because the duration of action of the antagonist is often shorter than the opiate, multiple doses may be required. Extreme caution must be employed when treating an addict with naloxone—a potentially severe withdrawal syndrome may ensue.

Ethylene glycol, a common component of automobile antifreeze, can cause death; this appears to be due to the production of specific metabolites. The treatment of acute ethylene glycol toxicity is similar to that used for other glycols and for methanol poisoning. While treating the metabolic acidosis with sodium bicarbonate, ethanol is used as a competitive substrate for alcohol dehydrogenase to reduce the formation of toxic metabolites.

Central Nervous System

DIRECTIONS: Each question below contains five suggested answers. Choose the **one best** response to each question.

183. The structure shown below is the parent compound of a group of compounds used primarily as

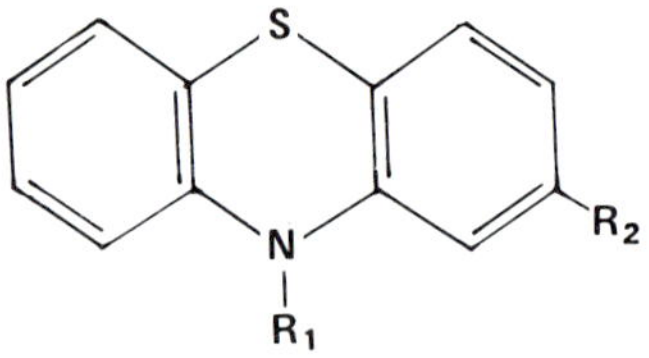

(A) anti-inflammatory agents
(B) antihypertensive agents
(C) major tranquilizers
(D) hypnotics
(E) tricyclic antidepressants

184. The use of morphine is contraindicated in which of the following situations?

(A) Myocardial infarction
(B) Cor pulmonale
(C) Dysentery
(D) Migraine headache
(E) Normal childbirth

185. An important action of metabolically demethylated imipramine is the blocking of

(A) norepinephrine release
(B) norepinephrine uptake
(C) dopamine release
(D) dopamine uptake
(E) serotonin synthesis

186. Which of the following statements about tricyclic antidepressants is correct?

(A) They have a mood-elevating effect when administered to a person whose health status is normal
(B) Their therapeutic effects become manifest after two to three weeks of administration
(C) They directly stimulate adrenergic receptors
(D) They have no significant cardiovascular effects
(E) They have weak anticholinergic effects

187. An extremely potent local anesthetic that may produce marked sedation is

(A) cocaine
(B) benzocaine
(C) procaine
(D) lidocaine
(E) tetracaine

188. Gingival hyperplasia is a complication of long-term antiepileptic treatment with

(A) phenobarbital (Luminal)
(B) primidone (Mysoline)
(C) trimethadione (Tridione)
(D) phenytoin (Dilantin)
(E) phensuximide (Milontin)

189. Physiological effects of alcohol intake include all the following EXCEPT

(A) sedation
(B) vasodilatation
(C) increased gastric secretion
(D) inhibition of the release of antidiuretic hormone
(E) increased cerebral blood flow

190. In selecting an antipsychotic agent for use in the treatment of a patient who has become psychotic for the first time, the most important characteristic of the drug to consider is its

(A) potency
(B) efficacy
(C) side effects
(D) rapidity of therapeutic action
(E) degree of lipid solubility

191. After intravenous injection of 5 to 10 mg of tubocurarine chloride, muscular relaxation is produced first in which of the following sites?

(A) Muscles of deglutition
(B) Extraocular muscles
(C) Skeletal muscles of the limbs
(D) Diaphragm
(E) Intestinal smooth muscle

192. A propensity to liver damage has been associated with repeated exposure to which of the following anesthetic agents?

(A) Ether
(B) Halothane
(C) Cyclopropane
(D) Nitrous oxide
(E) Morphine

193. The onset and duration of action of a barbiturate are mainly a function of its

(A) lipid solubility
(B) molecular weight
(C) plasma binding
(D) renal excretion
(E) method of administration

194. The first enzyme that acts to degrade ethanol is alcohol

(A) sulfatase
(B) reductase
(C) transferase
(D) dehydrogenase
(E) synthetase

195. Effects of major tranquilizers, like the phenothiazines, include all the following EXCEPT

(A) autonomic manifestations
(B) extrapyramidal manifestations
(C) anesthesia
(D) prevention of vomiting
(E) control of psychotic behavior

196. Which of the following statements about oral doses of chloral hydrate is true?

(A) They do not irritate the gastric mucosa
(B) They do not produce physical dependence
(C) They produce hypnosis rapidly
(D) They effectively produce analgesia
(E) They are metabolized by the hepatic microsomal enzyme system

197. Benzodiazepines have which of the following effects on the waking EEG?

(A) An increase in α activity
(B) A decrease in low-voltage fast activity
(C) A reduction of cortical somatosensory-evoked potentials
(D) A shift in activity evenly distributed over the entire brain
(E) A shift in activity from frontal to posterior regions of the brain

198. Diffusion hypoxia is most likely caused by which of the following inhalation anesthetics?

(A) Cyclopropane
(B) Enflurane
(C) Fluroxene
(D) Halothane
(E) Nitrous oxide

199. Carbidopa is useful in the treatment of Parkinson's disease because it

(A) is a precursor of L-dopa
(B) is a dopamine agonist
(C) prevents peripheral breakdown of L-dopa
(D) prevents breakdown of dopamine
(E) promotes regeneration of dopaminergic neurons

200. Chlorpromazine (Thorazine) is related structurally to all the following drugs EXCEPT

(A) chlordiazepoxide (Librium)
(B) perphenazine (Trilafon)
(C) procholorperazine (Compazine)
(D) thioridazine (Mellaril)
(E) trifluoperazine (Stelazine)

201. Grand mal or focal seizures are best treated with which of the following drugs?

(A) Chlorpromazine (Thorazine)
(B) Phenytoin (Dilantin)
(C) Paramethadione (Paradione)
(D) Phensuximide (Milontin)
(E) Thioridazine (Mellaril)

202. The preferred treatment of status epilepticus is intravenous administration of which of the following drugs?

(A) Chlorpromazine (Thorazine)
(B) Diazepam (Valium)
(C) Succinylcholine (Anectine)
(D) Tranylcypromine (Parnate)
(E) Trimethadione (Tridione)

203. There is substantial evidence that the important action of neuroleptic drugs is the blockade of the

(A) serotin receptor
(B) dopamine receptor
(C) γ-aminobutyric acid (GABA) receptor
(D) α-2 noradrenergic receptor
(E) glutamate receptor

204. The longest duration of action has been demonstrated with which one of the following barbiturates?

(A) Amobarbital (Amytal)
(B) Pentobarbital sodium (Nembutal)
(C) Phenobarbital (Luminal)
(D) Secobarbital sodium (Seconal)
(E) Thiopental sodium (Pentothal)

205. Flashback symptoms causing intense, incapacitating anxiety may occur in some patients who have abused

(A) ethanol
(B) secobarbital sodium (Seconal)
(C) diazepam (Valium)
(D) mescaline
(E) cocaine

206. Some antihistaminics have a marked sedative action in addition to their decongestant, antiurticaria, and antinausea properties. The greatest sedation is produced by which of the following antihistamines?

(A) Chlorpheniramine maleate (Chlor-Trimeton)
(B) Cyproheptadine ((Periactin)
(C) Tripelennamine (PBZ)
(D) Promethazine (Phenergan)
(E) Chlorothen (Tagathen)

207. Which of the following statements about cocaine is true?

(A) It potentiates the effects of injected epinephrine
(B) It blocks the action of acetylcholine
(C) It converts arrhythmias to normal sinus rhythms
(D) It is easily destroyed by plasma esterases
(E) It can be substituted clinically for quinidine

208. Sensitivity to barbiturates is greatest in which of the following areas of the central nervous system?

(A) Cortex
(B) Hypothalamus
(C) Limbic system
(D) Reticular activating system
(E) Spinal cord

209. To achieve field block anesthesia, a clinician must administer the local anesthetic in which of the following ways?

(A) By direct application to mucous membranes
(B) By injection into the lumbar subarachnoid space below the termination of the cord
(C) By injection into the tissue to be excised or mechanically stimulated
(D) By injection into or about individual peripheral nerves or nerve plexuses
(E) By injection to interrupt nerve transmission proximal to the site to be anesthetized

210. Which of the following statements about propoxyphene (Darvon) is true?

(A) It is related structurally to methadone
(B) It is subject to the same legal controls as morphine
(C) It is a more potent analgesic than codeine
(D) It does not suppress the withdrawal symptoms experienced by patients who are physically dependent on morphine or other narcotics
(E) It has a high abuse potential

211. The pharmacologic effects of morphine include all the following EXCEPT

(A) behavioral changes
(B) respiratory depression
(C) nausea
(D) diarrhea
(E) orthostatic hypotension

DIRECTIONS: Each question below contains four suggested answers of which **one** or **more** is correct. Choose the answer:

A	if	**1, 2, and 3**	are correct
B	if	**1 and 3**	are correct
C	if	**2 and 4**	are correct
D	if	**4**	is correct
E	if	**1, 2, 3, and 4**	are correct

212. Centrally acting muscle relaxants can be described as agents that

(1) are typified by chlordiazepoxide (Librium)
(2) produce flaccidity in therapeutic oral doses
(3) depress neuronal conduction and neuromuscular transmission
(4) are administered intravenously to treat acute muscle spasm

213. Opioid analgesics are often abused, causing severe social problems. True statements concerning opioid abuse include which of the following?

(1) Cross-tolerance develops for chemically dissimilar opioid analgesics
(2) Tolerance develops equally to all effects of opioids
(3) Opioids reduce pain, aggression, and sexual drives; their use is unlikely to induce crime if an adequate supply of the narcotic is available
(4) The quality of acute methadone withdrawal syndrome differs from that of acute heroin withdrawal

214. Phenobarbital, widely used in the control of tonic-clonic seizures, is associated with which of the following side effects?

(1) Extrapyramidal motor effects
(2) Nystagmus and ataxia
(3) Gingival hyperplasia
(4) Megaloblastic anemia

215. Benzodiazepine derivatives, such as chlordiazepoxide (Librium), have long been used in the treatment of anxiety. True statements concerning their use include which of the following?

(1) Their major locus of central depressant action is the brain stem reticular activating system
(2) They increase the seizure threshold
(3) Their prolonged use is associated with a physical dependence syndrome
(4) They are proven skeletal muscle relaxants

SUMMARY OF DIRECTIONS

A	B	C	D	E
1, 2, 3 only	1, 3 only	2, 4 only	4 only	All are correct

216. Pharmacologic properties of phenothiazine derivatives include an

(1) ability to produce weak antihistaminic effects
(2) absence of effect on the reuptake of γ-aminobutyric acid
(3) ability to prevent norepinephrine uptake by tissues
(4) ability to potentiate the effects of morphine

217. The CNS receives potent stimulation from which of the following agents?

(1) Caffeine
(2) Theobromine
(3) Theophylline
(4) Ethyl alcohol

218. Toxic, dose-related effects of the phenothiazines include which of the following?

(1) Parkinsonism
(2) Dystonia
(3) Akathisia
(4) Hyperpigmentation of the skin

219. Aspirin may be fatal if taken in sufficient quantity. The syndrome of acute aspirin overdose in children is characterized by

(1) marked hypothermia secondary to an antipyretic effect
(2) hypoglycemia
(3) peripheral edema
(4) disturbances in fluid and electrolyte balance

220. The pharmacologic properties of acetylsalicylic acid include an ability to

(1) produce in febrile, but rarely in nonfebrile, patients a rapid and effective reduction in temperature
(2) alleviate pain by both central nervous system and peripheral nervous system action
(3) alleviate low-intensity pain more effectively in peripheral than in visceral structures
(4) produce antipyrexia by a direct effect on hypothalamic neurons

221. Dextroamphetamine has actions that include

(1) elevation of the diastolic blood pressure
(2) reduction of fatigue and improvement in the performance of simple tasks
(3) less pronounced central effects and more pronounced peripheral effects than methamphetamine
(4) relaxation of bronchial muscle

222. Once equilibrium between an inhalation anesthetic in the inspired air and in the tissues is reached, the tissue concentration of the anesthetic is a function of the

(1) tissue blood flow
(2) lipid solubility of the anesthetic
(3) tissue P_{O_2}
(4) concentration of the anesthetic in the inspired air

223. Patients receiving a monoamine oxidase inhibitor are subject to strict dietary restrictions. Such restrictions involve a prohibition of

(1) aged cheeses
(2) beer
(3) pickled herring
(4) wine

224. Side effects of chlorpromazine (Thorazine) include

(1) palpitations
(2) orthostatic hypotension
(3) blood dyscrasias
(4) obstructive jaundice

225. One of the most beneficial drugs in the treatment of Parkinson's disease is the recently developed L-dopa. The drug exhibits peculiar interactions with other drugs and merits precautionary measures in certain situations. True statements concerning L-dopa include which of the following?

(1) L-Dopa has been associated with increased growth of melanoma
(2) Pyridoxine, in the doses found in over-the-counter multivitamin preparations, will reverse the therapeutic effects of L-dopa
(3) Marked hypertension may occur when L-dopa is used in conjunction with monoamine oxidase inhibitors
(4) L-Dopa is contraindicated in patients with narrow-angle glaucoma

226. Drugs that are especially useful in the treatment of petit mal epilepsy include

(1) phenobarbital
(2) trimethadione
(3) carbamazepine
(4) ethosuximide

227. Plant alkaloids that are derived from the poppy plant *Papaver somniferum* include

(1) morphine
(2) papaverine
(3) codeine
(4) muscarine

228. Substances with marked antipsychotic properties can be found within which of the following classes of compounds?

(1) Butyrophenones
(2) Phenothiazines
(3) Thioxanthenes
(4) Benzodiazepines

229. Correct statements concerning hydroxyzine, an antianxiety agent, include which of the following?

(1) It causes drug disposition tolerance
(2) It induces sleep in large doses
(3) It binds to benzodiazepine receptors
(4) It is an antihistaminic agent

230. Benefits of preanesthetic medications include their ability to

(1) increase the effectiveness of an incomplete anesthetic
(2) decrease the dosage of anesthetic needed
(3) counteract undesirable side effects of anesthetic agents
(4) relieve anxiety

SUMMARY OF DIRECTIONS

A	B	C	D	E
1, 2, 3 only	1, 3 only	2, 4 only	4 only	All are correct

231. True statements concerning the tricyclic antidepressants include which of the following?

(1) The central ring is characterized by an ethylene linkage
(2) They may have serious cardiotoxic effects
(3) They are inactivated as a result of ultimate conjugation with glucuronic acid
(4) They can increase anxiety in normal subjects

232. Patients being treated with phenobarbital and phenytoin for epilepsy may experience which of the following untoward effects?

(1) Skin rash
(2) Gingival hyperplasia
(3) Lupus erythematosus-like syndrome
(4) Fever

233. An abstinence syndrome indicating physical dependence or addiction occurs with the acute withdrawal of

(1) morphine
(2) ethanol
(3) phenobarbital
(4) chlorpromazine

234. Correct statements concerning special slow-releasing preparations of barbiturates include which of the following?

(1) They are used to circumvent the problem of short half-lives of these drugs
(2) They are used in hypnotic therapy
(3) They are used as substitutes for benzodiazepines
(4) They are potentially dangerous

235. The antidepressant effect of tranylcypromine (Parnate) can be attributed to

(1) a direct nicotine-like stimulation
(2) a direct amphetamine-like stimulation
(3) a xanthine-like stimulant effect
(4) the inhibition of monoamine oxidase

236. Local anesthetics, like general anesthetics, produce

(1) analgesia
(2) relaxation
(3) hyporeflexia
(4) narcosis

237. Consequences of prolonged, excessive use of ethyl alcohol include

(1) possible development of tolerance
(2) heightened sensitivity to barbiturates experienced only by an **intoxicated** alcoholic person
(3) possible development of a life-threatening withdrawal syndrome when consumption of alcohol is abruptly ended
(4) possible development of malnutrition

238. The hypnotic or anesthetic potency of barbiturates is influenced by which of the following physical and physiologic properties?

(1) Rate of entry into the brain as compared with other tissues
(2) Rate of metabolism and excretion
(3) Ionization potential
(4) Water solubility

239. Correct statements concerning fentanyl, a synthetic opioid related to the phenylpiperidines, include which of the following?

(1) It is used almost exclusively for anesthesia
(2) It has been shown to be 80 times more potent than morphine
(3) It produces muscular rigidity at high doses that is reversed by naloxone
(4) Its analgesic effects are intensified by droperidol

240. Halothane, the most popular anesthetic agent in the western hemisphere, has characteristics that include

(1) high lipid solubility
(2) ability to cause respiratory depression with increased anesthetic depth
(3) possible hepatotoxicity
(4) ability to increase cardiac output

241. Drugs used for the treatment of Parkinson's disease include

(1) L-dopa
(2) trihexyphenidyl (Tremin)
(3) amantadine (Symmetrel)
(4) reserpine (Serpasil)

242. Characteristics of lithium carbonate include

(1) a general sedative action similar to that of the phenothiazine tranquilizers
(2) a relatively late peak plasma level, which occurs 16 to 24 hours after ingestion
(3) a toxicity level approaching 50% substitution of plasma sodium ion, (about 50-80 mEq/L)
(4) a controlling effect on both mania and depression

243. Moderate doses of morphine have which of the following effects on a normal resting individual?

(1) Respiratory depression
(2) Increased biliary tract pressure
(3) Pruritus and sweating
(4) Decreased cardiac output

244. Correct statements about tardive dyskinesia resulting from major tranquilizer therapy include which of the following?

(1) It is a condition of impaired control over voluntary oral and facial muscles
(2) It has symptoms that often occur after the therapy ends
(3) It often persists as a permanent condition in elderly institutionalized patients
(4) It is a condition that responds favorably to treatment with L-dopa

DIRECTIONS: The groups of questions below consist of lettered choices followed by several numbered items. For each numbered item select the **one** lettered choice with which it is **most** closely associated. Each lettered choice may be used once, more than once, or not at all.

Questions 245-248

For each of the following descriptions, select the drug with which it is most closely associated.

(A) Ethosuximide
(B) Phenytoin
(C) Carbamazepine
(D) Dipropylacetate
(E) Diazepam

245. Drug of choice in petit mal

246. May act by elevating γ-aminobutyric acid levels in the brain

247. Drug of choice in status epilepticus for immediate action

248. Structurally and pharmacologically similar to the hydantoins

Questions 249-252

For each of the following descriptions, select the drug with which it is most closely associated.

(A) Chloral hydrate
(B) Thiopental
(C) Phenobarbital
(D) Flurazepam
(E) Phenytoin

249. Contraindicated in acute intermittent porphyria

250. Long-acting because of psychoactive metabolites

251. Undergoes enzymatic reduction to an active metabolite

252. Extremely short-acting due to rapid redistribution

Questions 253-257

Many drugs are associated with an ability to induce physical dependence as well as a craving for the tolerance to their psychological effects. For each of the drugs listed below, choose the effect that it usually produces.

(A) Craving only
(B) Craving and tolerance
(C) Tolerance and physical dependence
(D) Craving, tolerance, and physical dependence
(E) None of the above

253. Cocaine

254. Heroin

255. Amphetamine

256. Secobarbital

257. Chlorpromazine

Central Nervous System
Answers

183. The answer is C. *(Gilman, ed 6. pp 396, 408.)* The parent compound of the phenothiazines, a class of agents primarily used as major tranquilizers, consists of two benzene rings linked by a sulfur and nitrogen atom to form a three-ring structure as shown in the question. It is similar to anthracene, except that C 9 is replaced by sulfur, C 10 is replaced by nitrogen, and various groups (R_1 and R_2) are substituents on the nitrogen and C 3 of the generic phenothiazine molecule, as depicted in the following structures:

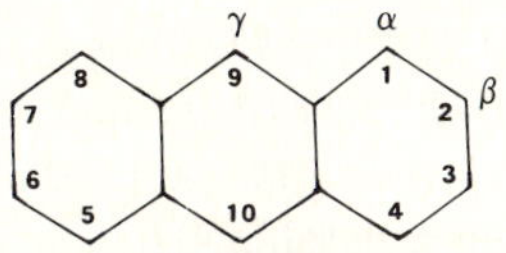
Anthracene

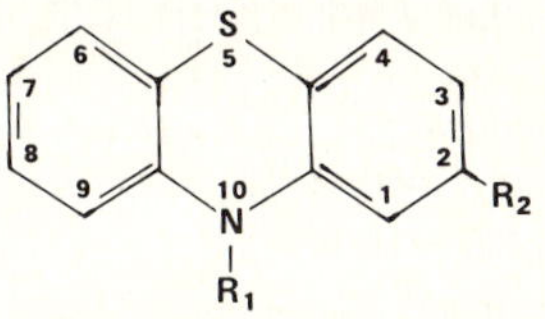
Phenothiazine Parent Compound

If R_2 is chlorine, the potency for depressing motor activity is increased. If R_2 is a piperazine or piperazinyl group, the parent compound becomes the most potent of the phenothiazine antipsychotic drugs. Tricyclic antidepressants have an ethylene bridge as a replacement for the sulfur and have no substitutions at R_2.

184. The answer is B. *(Gilman, ed 6. pp 508, 511-513.)* Deaths have occurred from the administration of therapeutic doses of morphine to patients who had cor pulmonale (pulmonary heart disease). For patients who have coronary artery disease, morphine can be beneficial because it decreases oxygen consumption and cardiac work. Morphine reduces the peristaltic contractions of the gastrointestinal tract and thus is useful in treating patients who have dysentery. Therapeutic doses of morphine do not affect cerebral circulation and the normally contracting uterus.

185. The answer is B. *(Gilman, ed 6. p 421.)* Imipramine, a tricyclic antidepressant, blocks the neuronal uptake of norepinephrine and serotonin. Thus, the effect of sympathomimetic amines that act directly is enhanced by tricyclic antidepressants. The demethylated metabolites are believed to have a particular specificity for norepinephrine uptake, and to limit both hormonal secretion and the rate at which adrenergic neurons in the locus ceruleus are fired.

186. The answer is B. *(Gilman, ed 6. pp 419-421.)* Patients who are receiving tricyclic antidepressants should be informed that 2 to 3 weeks must pass before the therapeutic effects of the drug are evident. Patients who are not depressed feel drowsy—but do not experience euphoria or mood-elevation—after taking these drugs. Tricyclic antidepressants do not stimulate adrenergic receptors but block the reuptake of norepinephrine and serotonin into nerve terminals. These drugs have a tendency to produce cardiac arrhythmias. In addition, tricyclic antidepressants have been reported to cause anticholinergic side effects (such as dry mouth, blurred vision, constipation, and urinary retention) in both normal and depressed patients.

187. The answer is D. *(Gilman, ed 6. pp 308-309.)* Local anesthetics are drugs that, when applied locally, block nerve conduction; they also prevent generation of the nerve impulse. When injected, lidocaine produces more prompt, more intense, and longer lasting anesthesia than do equivalent doses of the other agents listed in the question. Sleepiness and a possibly metabolite-induced dizziness are frequent side effects of lidocaine.

188. The answer is D. *(Gilman, ed 6. p 454.)* Adverse or toxic effects resulting from administration of phenytoin (Dilantin) are related to the route and duration of exposure and to dosage. Approximately 20 percent of patients receiving phenytoin on a chronic basis suffer gingival hyperplasia; in young adolescents and children, it is the most frequent toxic manifestation of this drug. Osteomalacia, megaloblastic anemia, hirsutism, and cerebellar-vestibular effects are other adverse effects associated with phenytoin therapy.

189. The answer is E. *(Gilman, ed 6. pp 376-386.)* Alcohol, commonly regarded by the laity as a stimulant, is a primary and continuous depressant of the central nervous system. In moderate doses, alcohol produces cutaneous vasodilatation; however, there is no change in cerebral blood flow, cerebral metabolism, or cerebrovascular resistance. Gastric and salivary secretions are stimulated. Diuresis occurs secondary to inhibition of posterior pituitary antidiuretic hormone.

190. The answer is C. *(Gilman, ed 6. pp 414-415.)* In the treatment of psychotic persons, the selection of an antipsychotic agent rests largely upon its side effects, owing to the lack of therapeutic specificity characteristic of this class of drugs. The effectiveness of a particular drug or combination of drugs on a symptom complex is chiefly a matter of trial and error. A patient with a history of cardiovascular disease or stroke should be given the smallest effective dose.

191. The answer is B. *(Gilman, ed 6. p 226.)* Curare-induced muscular relaxation first appears in small rapidly moving muscles, such as those of the fingers, toes, eyes, and ears, and then in the muscles of the limbs, neck, and trunk. Ultimately, the intercostal muscles—and finally the diaphragm—are paralyzed, and respiration ceases.

192. The answer is B. *(Gilman, ed 6. p 282.)* Hepatic damage has been reported to occur following halothane anesthesia, although the incidence is low. Repeated exposure to halothane apparently increases the likelihood of hepatic damage, which is distinguished by extensive hepatocellular necrosis that is predominantly centrilobular in location. The reaction is believed to be allergic in character.

193. The answer is A. *(Gilman, ed 6. pp 351-358.)* In general, structural changes that increase the lipid solubility of barbiturates will decrease the duration of action, hasten the onset of activity, accelerate metabolic degradation, and often increase hypnotic potency.

194. The answer is D. *(Gilman, ed 6. p 383.)* Of all the alcohol that enters the body, 90 to 98 percent is completely oxidized. Initial oxidation, which occurs chiefly in the liver, involves conversion of alcohol to acetaldehyde by alcohol dehydrogenase. The acetaldehyde is then converted to acetyl CoA, which enters the Krebs cycle or participates in a variety of anabolic synthetic reactions.

195. The answer is C. *(Gilman, ed 6. pp 398-404.)* The tranquilizers listed in the question are sedatives; by themselves they do not produce anesthesia. Autonomic and extrapyramidal motor effects commonly result from use of these drugs, probably due to adrenergic and dopaminergic blocking actions. Major tranquilizers such as phenothiazines are used primarily to control psychotic behavior. Although effective against vomiting produced by some drugs and disease states, they are not effective for control of motion sickness.

196. The answer is C. *(Gilman, ed 6. pp 362-363.)* Oral doses of chloral hydrate rapidly produce hypnosis and may cause epigastric distress, nausea, and vomiting. Although not metabolized by the hepatic microsomal system, chloral hydrate accelerates the metabolism of some drugs that are metabolized by this system. Habitual use of chloral hydrate can lead to physical dependence and delirium when the drug is withdrawn. Like the barbiturates, it has little analgesic activity and may produce excitement in the presence of pain.

197. The answer is C. *(Gilman, ed 6. p 342.)* In the waking EEG, benzodiazepines diminish the amplitude of somatosensory-evoked potentials. This results in a shortening in the latency of the early peak and a prolonging of the late peak, changes that, together with a shift to β activity, are believed to be responsible for the antianxiety actions of these drugs.

198. The answer is E. *(Goth, ed 10. pp 264-265.)* The large volume of nitrous oxide, N_2O, dissolved in the blood moves back into the alveoli by simple diffusion when administration of the gas is stopped. Thus, the alveolar concentration of oxygen may, temporarily, be markedly depressed. This situation is referred to as diffusion hypoxia.

199. The answer is C. *(Gilman, ed 6. p 482.)* Carbidopa is an inhibitor of L-dopa decarboxylase that cannot readily move into the CNS and decreases the decarboxylation of L-dopa in the peripheral tissues. These effects promote an increased concentration of L-dopa in the nigrostriatum, where the receptors are located.

200. The answer is A. *(Goth, ed 10. pp 283-284, 289.)* Chlordiazepoxide (Librium) is a benzodiazepine antianxiety drug; the other drugs listed in the question all contain the phenothiazine nucleus and may be considered major tranquilizers. The benzodiazepines prevent chemically induced convulsions; phenothiazines do not. Benzodiazepines have no significant extrapyramidal or autonomic side effects.

201. The answer is B. *(Goth, ed 10. pp 283, 335-338.)* Of the drugs listed in the question, phenytoin (Dilantin) is preferred for treatment of persons who have grand mal or focal seizures. Hydantoins, barbiturates, and carbonic anhydrase inhibitors also may be used to control grand mal epilepsy. Chlorpromazine (Thorazine) and thioridazine (Mellaril) are antipsychotic drugs, which do not affect grand mal epilepsy. Paramethadione (Paradione) and phensuximide (Milontin) are useful in petit mal epilepsy but are not generally used in grand mal seizures.

202. The answer is B. *(Goth, ed 10. p 338.)* Intravenously administered diazepam (Valium) is the drug of choice for treatment of status epilepticus. It has been suggested that diazepam increases the apparent affinity of the inhibitory neurotransmitter γ-aminobutyric acid (GABA) for binding sites on brain cell membranes. None of the other drugs listed in the question is appropriate for status epilepticus: chlorpromazine (Thorazine) is a major tranquilizer; succinylcholine (Anectine) is a neuromuscular blocking agent; tranylcypromine (Parnate) is an antidepressant; trimethadione (Tridione) is used in petit mal epilepsy.

203. The answer is B. *(Gilman, ed 6. p 401.)* Relatively small amounts of neuroleptic drugs have been shown to interfere with the effects of dopaminergic agonists. They also increase the rate of production of dopamine antagonists. Specifically, it has been demonstrated that a selective dopamine-sensitive adenylate cyclase system present in caudate or limbic tissues is inhibited by these drugs.

204. The answer is C. *(Goth, ed 10. p 304.)* Phenobarbital sodium (Luminal) is classed as a long-acting barbiturate. Thiopental is a short-acting, intravenously administered barbiturate. Secobarbital and pentobarbital are short-acting, orally administered barbiturates; amobarbital is classed as an intermediate-acting barbiturate. It should be noted, however, that this classification of barbiturates does not necessarily correspond to their clinical effectiveness in producing sleep.

205. The answer is D. *(Goth, ed 10. pp 378, 380.)* Flashback symptoms occur most frequently with abuse of psychotomimetics, such as LSD, STP, tryptamines, mescaline, or morning glory seeds. Patients reported that these symptoms often continue to occur as late as one year after the last dose.

206. The answer is D. *(Goth, ed 10. p 251.)* Of the antihistaminics listed in the question, promethazine (Phenergan) has the greatest—and chlorothen (Tagathen) the least—sedative action. In an acute situation, Phenergan is usually given intramuscularly. Sedation can be an undesirable side effect when these drugs are used orally to control motion sickness or allergic rhinitis. Tagathen is not currently available.

207. The answer is A. *(Gilman, ed 6. pp 307-308.)* Cocaine is known to interfere with the uptake of norepinephrine by adrenergic nerve terminals and to potentiate both the excitatory and inhibitory responses of sympathetically innervated organs to epinephrine, norepinephrine, and sympathetic nerve stimulation. Cocaine is metabolized by the liver, although some of the drug may be excreted unchanged in urine. It is used clinically as a surface anesthetic agent.

208. The answer is D. *(Gilman, ed 6. pp 352-355.)* Barbiturates depress activity at all levels of the neuraxis, or central nervous system. However, the reticular activating system is particularly sensitive to barbiturates and other sedative-hypnotics, and it appears that depression of this system is responsible for the sedation induced by these drugs. Nevertheless, pain sensation remains intact until barbiturate blood levels are sufficient to induce unconsciousness.

209. The answer is E. *(Gilman, ed 6. p 312.)* Field block anesthesia, as compared to infiltration anesthesia, affords a greater area of anesthetization with less drug. This technique is notably advantageous for anesthesia of the scalp, anterior abdominal wall, and leg. Success with this procedure requires a more than passing acquaintance with regional neuroanatomy.

210. The answer is A. *(Gilman, ed 6. pp 520-522.)* The structure of propoxyphene hydrochloride (Darvon) is very similar to that of methadone. Propoxyphene, unlike pentazocine lactate (Talwin), another synthetic narcotic, has no antagonistic activity and thus does not precipitate withdrawal. Because of its relatively low abuse potential, propoxyphene is not as tightly controlled as morphine or methadone. It is about one-third as potent as codeine.

211. The answer is D. *(Gilman, ed 6. pp 499-505.)* Morphine decreases the motility of the stomach and the propulsive contractions of the small and large intestines, thereby producing constipation. It can produce euphoric or dysphoric reactions, depending on the personality of the patient and the setting in which it is administered. Respiratory depression is the major cause of death associated with morphine overdoses. Orthostatic hypotension and nausea are common in ambulatory patients.

212. **The answer is D (4).** *(Gilman, ed 6. pp 488-491.)* The treatment of acute muscle spasm by intravenous administration of centrally acting muscle relaxants is well-established. These drugs do not depress neuronal conduction or neuromuscular transmission, as does curare. Instead, they depress spinal polysynaptic reflexes. Flaccidity is not the action produced by administration of therapeutically appropriate oral doses. The antianxiety agent chlordiazepoxide does not have enough muscle-relaxant potency to be useful for this purpose; its benefit in muscle tension associated with anxiety is derived from its sedative properties.

213. **The answer is B (1, 3).** *(Gilman, ed 6. pp 505, 546-548.)* In opioid abuse, there is always a high degree of cross-tolerance to other drugs with a similar pharmacologic action even if the chemical composition of the opioids is totally different. Tolerance develops at different rates to different effects of opioids. With methadone, abrupt withdrawal causes a syndrome that is qualitatively similar to that of morphine but is longer and less intense, thus following the general rule that a drug with a shorter duration of action produces a shorter, more intense withdrawal syndrome. The crimes associated with narcotic abuse are considered to be motivated by the need to **acquire** the drug and not from the effects of the drug per se.

214. **The answer is C (2, 4).** *(Gilman, ed 6. pp 406, 454, 457.)* Excessive doses of phenobarbital may result in nystagmus and ataxia. Folate-responsive megaloblastic anemia is a less common side effect. Phenytoin, the other widely used drug for control of tonic-clonic seizures, is known for its ability to produce gingival hyperplasia. Extrapyramidal side effects are characteristic of major tranquilizers such as the phenothiazines, which are ineffective against seizures.

215. **The answer is A (1, 2, 3).** *(Gilman, ed 6. pp 347-348.)* All benzodiazepine compounds increase seizure threshold and are effective anticonvulsant agents. These drugs block EEG arousal from stimulation of the brain stem reticular formation. Tolerance and physical dependence occur with benzodiazepines, but very high doses must be given before marked withdrawal symptoms appear. Although the drugs are widely used clinically as skeletal muscle relaxants, controlled studies have not proven their advantage over placebo administration.

216. The answer is E (all). *(Gilman, ed 6. pp 397-404.)* Phenothiazine derivatives, such as chlorpromazine, prevent the reuptake of norepinephrine and 5-hydroxytryptamine in laboratory animals but do not affect the reuptake of γ-aminobutyric acid, or piperidinic acid. These drugs exhibit peripheral cholinergic and α-adrenergic blocking activity, adrenergic activity, and antihistaminic and antitryptaminergic activity. Chlorpromazine has been shown to increase the miotic and sedative effects of morphine. Indeed, the phenothiazines markedly affect the actions of numerous drugs.

217. The answer is B (1, 3). *(Gilman, ed 6. pp 376, 592-593.)* The xanthines caffeine and theophylline are potent stimulators of the CNS. The related xanthine, theobromine, is virtually ineffective in this respect. Despite the popular view of alcohol as a "stimulant," it is incontrovertibly a CNS depressant.

218. The answer is E (all). *(Gilman, ed 6. pp 407, 413.)* Abnormal skin pigmentation can result from long-term administration of the phenothiazines in high doses. The reaction manifests itself as a slate gray pigmentation in sun-exposed skin areas. A parkinsonian syndrome identical to idiopathic parkinsonism may also develop with therapy. Other toxic effects of the phenothiazines include akathisia, or a compulsion to be in constant motion, and acute dystonic reactions manifested by facial grimacing or torticollis.

219. The answer is C (2, 4). *(Gilman, ed 6. p 696.)* The most prominent feature of salicylate intoxication in children is a combination of respiratory acidosis and metabolic acidosis—a situation that constitutes a medical emergency. Hypoglycemia may also be a serious consequence of a salicylate overdose. Hyperthermia and dehydration are the immediate threats to life, and initial therapy is directed toward correction of these parameters. Aspirin, in large doses, increases oxygen consumption and metabolic rate.

220. The answer is A (1, 2, 3). *(Gilman, ed 6. pp 689-690.)* Aspirin (acetylsalicylic acid), the most extensively used analgesic, antipyretic, and anti-inflammatory agent, acts generally by virtue of its salicylic acid content. The antipyretic effect and the analgesic effect appear to involve the inhibition of the synthesis of prostaglandins and their effects on the hypothalamus and local sites. Low-intensity pain generated from integumentary structures responds to aspirin, whereas visceral pain usually does not.

221. The answer is E (all). *(Gilman, ed 6. pp 160, 162.)* An oral dose of dextroamphetamine raises both systolic and diastolic blood pressures. The effects of fatigue are reduced in the short-run, and the performance of simple or repetitive tasks is enhanced. The pharmacologic actions of dextroamphetamine and methamphetamine are similar, but the ratio of central to peripheral actions is different. Bronchial smooth muscle is relaxed—but not sufficiently to be therapeutically useful.

222. The answer is D (4). *(Gilman, ed 6. pp 260-263.)* Pulmonary ventilation, blood flow, and agent solubility in blood and tissue affect both the uptake and elimination of inhalation anesthetic agents. When equilibrium between arterial tension and inspired tension has been reached, changes in inspired air concentration are followed by changes in arterial blood tension, which results in changes in tissue concentration.

223. The answer is E (all). *(Gilman, ed 6. pp 204-205.)* All the foods and beverages listed in the question (and other foods) contain tyramine, which releases norepinephrine. Because hepatic monoamine oxidase (MAO) is inhibited in patients receiving MAO inhibitors, tyramine escapes oxidative deamination and releases supranormal amounts of norepinephrine from nerve endings. The result can be a severe hypertensive crisis culminating in intracranial bleeding and death.

224. The answer is E (all). *(Gilman, ed 6. pp 406-407, 413.)* Phenothiazines are usually regarded as safe agents. At therapeutic doses, however, side effects such as palpitations and orthostatic hypotension can occur. Blood dyscrasias may appear suddenly and are potentially very dangerous. Obstructive jaundice is a hypersensitivity reaction occurring in 2 to 4 percent of patients receiving phenothiazines.

225. The answer is E (all). *(Gilman, ed 6. p 481.)* Administration of supplemental pyridoxine increases decarboxylase activity, thus more L-dopa is converted to dopamine in the periphery and less is available for central nervous system penetration. Use of monoamine oxidase inhibitors is contraindicated in patients taking L-dopa because hypertension may result. Patients with known melanomas or pigmented lesions should be carefully watched because L-dopa therapy has been associated with increased growth of melanoma. Narrow-angle glaucoma is a definite contraindication to L-dopa therapy, and wide-angle glaucoma must be monitored by repeated measurements of intraocular pressure.

226. The answer is C (2, 4). *(Gilman, ed 6. pp 461, 464-465.)* Both ethosuximide and trimethadione are used to treat petit mal epilepsy. Because ethosuximide is more effective than trimethadione against absence seizures and exhibits fewer serious adverse effects, it is the agent of choice for this type of epilepsy. Carbamazepine is effective in the treatment of temporal lobe epilepsy. Phenobarbital is an effective agent for generalized tonic-clonic and cortical focal seizures.

227. The answer is A (1, 2, 3). *(Gilman, ed 6. pp 98, 494-495.)* Heroin and a score of clinically useful alkaloids, including morphine, papaverine, and codeine, are derived from the poppy seed. Muscarine, the cause of mushroom poisoning or mycetismus, is found in *Amanita muscaria* and various species of *Inocybe*.

228. The answer is A (1, 2, 3). *(Gilman, ed 6. pp 408-411, 440.)* The most prominent member of the butyrophenones is the antipsychotic drug haloperidol. Chlorpromazine is a phenothiazine, and chlorprothixene belongs to the thioxanthene family. Benzodiazepines, such as diazepam, have antianxiety, but not antipsychotic, properties.

229. The answer is C (2, 4). *(Gilman, ed 6. p 269.)* Hydroxyzine is widely used as a preanesthetic medication. It is an antihistaminic, with sedation as one of its side effects, especially in high doses. Hydroxyzine only slightly depresses circulatory and respiratory functions and has no effect on the duration of anesthesia.

230. The answer is E (all). *(Goth, ed 10. pp 418-419.)* A variety of drugs is used before and during the administration of anesthetics in operative procedures, for all the reasons listed in the question. The most commonly used preanesthetic medications include narcotics, sedatives, hypnotics, antiemetics, and anticholinergics. Because of the many disadvantages associated with their use, preanesthetic drugs must be employed with care.

231. The answer is E (all). *(Gilman, ed 6. pp 419-423.)* The tricyclic antidepressants are structurally distinguished from the phenothiazines by substitution of an ethylene for a sulfur linkage in the central ring. In normal persons, the drugs' effects are usually perceived as unpleasant, resulting in a feeling of unhappiness and an increase in anxiety. Toxic reactions to the tricyclics include antimuscarinic, cerebral, and cardiac effects, especially in patients with cardiovascular disease.

232. The answer is E (all). *(Goth, ed 10. p 336.)* All the side effects listed in the question can occur as a result of antiepileptic therapy with phenobarbital and phenytoin. These potential toxic manifestations should be kept in mind so that a patient's treatment can be appropriately modified early in the course of therapy if such adverse effects occur.

233. The answer is A (1, 2, 3). *(Goth, ed 10. p 359.)* Physical dependence occurs following prolonged abuse of morphine, ethanol, and barbiturates. Acute withdrawal of these substances produces an abstinence syndrome, the severity of which depends upon the drug that was abused. Such a syndrome is not associated with the abuse of phenothiazine antipsychotic drugs like chlorpromazine.

234. The answer is D (4). *(Gilman, ed 6. pp 357, 361.)* Barbiturates have essentially been replaced by the benzodiazepines in all but a few special cases. Because the barbiturates have long half-lives (only 20 percent of an oral hypnotic dose of barbital is eliminated in the urine of normal adults in the first 24 hours), the use of slow-releasing forms is pointless and dangerous. Owing to the relatively high doses required for hypnotic use, these forms are particularly disadvantageous.

235. The answer is C (2, 4). *(Goth, ed 10. pp 293-294.)* Tranylcypromine (Parnate), a bimodal antidepressant, is a structural analog of amphetamine and has a rapid amphetamine-like stimulant effect. Over a longer period of time, tranylcypromine is a stimulant on the basis of its inhibition of monoamine oxidase, like iproniazid (Marsilid). The latter agent is not currently listed as an officially available drug under its generic or proprietary name.

236. The answer is A (1, 2, 3). *(Goth, ed 10. pp 431-432, 434.)* Local anesthetics are used to produce a reversible and short-lived loss of sensation in a localized area. Mechanistically, they interfere with the rate of rise of the depolarization phase of the action potential. Blockade of nerve fibers results in relaxation, loss of tone, and loss of sensation. Local anesthesia usually does not produce central nervous system effects.

237. The answer is E (all). *(Goth, ed 10. pp 363-364.)* Long-term, excessive consumption of alcohol will cause hypertrophy of the hepatic smooth endoplasmic reticulum, with a resultant increase in metabolism and, thus, tolerance. Barbiturates are metabolized via the same route; however, in the presence of alcohol, which is preferentially metabolized, they remain active longer. Alcohol withdrawal symptoms may be fatal. Alcohol supplies calories, depressing appetite and encouraging an inadequate diet in the face of a deceptive maintenance of body weight.

238. The answer is E (all). *(Goth, ed 10. p 305.)* Ideally, the most potent barbiturate should exhibit low water solubility, weak ionization, high oil-water partition coefficient, rapid entry into brain tissue, volume of distribution similar to that of total body water, and a rate of metabolism and excretion that is slow enough to allow the drug to reach its site of action in an effective concentration.

239. The answer is A (1, 2, 3). *(Gilman, ed 6. pp 295, 518.)* The synthetic opioid fentanyl is 80 times more potent than morphine and has a major use in anesthesia. Muscular rigidity produced by fentanyl very likely results from opioid influence on dopaminergic transmission in the striatum, an influence that is antagonized by naloxone. Droperidol neither strengthens nor sensibly prolongs the actions of fentanyl. The two agents are used together in intravenous anesthesia.

240. The answer is A (1, 2, 3). *(Goth, ed 10. p 425.)* The high solubility of halothane in blood and fat allows for the maintenance of anesthetic blood levels for prolonged periods. The death rate associated with halothane is similar to or slightly lower than that of other anesthetic agents. Hepatotoxicity does occasionally occur and appears to increase in incidence with increased exposure to halothane. Depression of respiratory centers expressed as a decreased ventilatory response to carbon dioxide occurs as anesthetic depth increases. Arterial hypotension and a reduction in cardiac output, peripheral resistance, and myocardial contractility occur at surgical levels of anesthesia.

241. The answer is A (1, 2, 3). *(Gilman, ed 6. pp 484-487.)* Although the first three drugs listed in the question are all used in the treatment of Parkinson's disease, L-dopa is the drug of choice. L-Dopa is a precursor of dopamine and crosses the blood-brain barrier. Its mechanism of action is thought to be replenishment of dopamine stores in the corpus striatum. Amantadine (Symmetrel) causes the release of dopamine from intact striatal neurons. Trihexyphenidyl (Tremin) is typical of the anticholinergic drugs that were used before L-dopa was introduced and is still occasionally beneficial in patients who have minimal symptoms. Reserpine (Serpasil), a major tranquilizer, is ineffective in the treatment of Parkinson's disease.

242. The answer is D (4). *(Gilman, ed 6. pp 431-432, 434.)* Lithium salts help to prevent and control mood swings in both manic and depressive directions. Unlike the major tranquilizers, lithium is not a sedative. It has an early peak plasma level at two to four hours after ingestion, and its toxicity level can be as low as 2 mEq/L.

243. The answer is A (1, 2, 3). *(Gilman, ed 6. pp 499-504.)* Morphine causes varying degrees of respiratory depression that are dose-related. Biliary tract pressure is markedly increased by morphine. Pruritus and sweating are common and probably result from histamine release. Morphine has little or no effect on the myocardium, heart rate, or cardiac output and thus can be given to patients who have myocardial infarcts.

244. The answer is A (1, 2, 3). *(Gilman, ed 6. pp 407, 412.)* The most prominent symptoms of tardive dyskinesia are involuntary tongue protrusions and lip-smacking. This condition is usually masked by major tranquilizer use; it appears when therapy is halted or the dosage reduced. Tardive dyskinesia is most common in elderly institutionalized patients, in whom the condition is usually permanent. It does not respond to L-dopa or any other antiparkinsonian drug; in fact, there is no generally accepted therapy.

245-248. The answers are: 245-A, 246-D, 247-E, 248-C. *(Gilman, ed 6. pp 459-464, 466-467.)* Ethosuximide and trimethadione exhibit similar anticonvulsant properties in animals. Both agents prevent pentylenetetrazol-induced convulsions. Ethosuximide also boosts the threshold for electroshock seizures and is the primary drug for treating absence seizures (petit mal).

Dipropylacetate (valproic acid), a recently developed antiepileptic agent, may act by increasing γ-aminobutyric acid (GABA) levels through a suppression of either GABA transaminase or of succinic semialdehyde dehydrogenase; it is also possible that GABA levels are increased by inhibition of reuptake by glial cells or nerve endings. Dipropylacetate is effective against many types of seizures, and its CNS side effects are trivial.

Although used chiefly for its antianxiety properties, diazepam has been important in managing status epilepticus; the drug must be administered intravenously in the treatment of seizure disorders. Based on the ability of benzodiazepines to increase the apparent affinity of GABA for binding site in brain membranes, it has been suggested that diazepam enhances the potency of GABA.

Carbamazepine exhibits considerable structural overlap with the hydantoins such as phenytoin. Its anticonvulsant effects in animals are also similar to phenytoin. Carbamazepine is generally useful for the treatment of trigeminal neuralgia. It has a number of serious side effects, including bone marrow depression and cardiovascular complications.

249-252. The answers are: 249-C, 250-D, 251-A, 252-B. *(Gilman, ed 6. pp 347, 357-358, 363.)* Phenobarbital and other barbiturates are known to stimulate porphyrin synthesis. For this reason, they should not be administered under any circumstances to patients with porphyria variegata or acute intermittent porphyria. Other important side effects of phenobarbital are paradoxical excitement, hypersensitivity, and residual depression.

Flurazepam and other benzodiazepines undergo a variety of biotransformations. The nonconjugated metabolites that are produced are also biologically active and result in a prolonged duration of action. This also results in complex pharmacokinetics.

Chloral hydrate undergoes enzymatic reduction to trichloroethanol, presumably in the liver as a consequence of alcohol dehydrogenase. This reaction is promoted by ethanol, oxidation of which enhances the reduction of chloral hydrate via NADH formation. The pharmacologic properties of trichloroethanol are essentially identical to those of chloral hydrate.

Thiopental, a highly lipid-soluble barbiturate, is rapidly taken up in the portions of the brain with the most generous blood supply, usually in the first 30 seconds. In the next 30 minutes the drug reaches the other portions of the brain, by which time the gray matter retains barely 10 percent of the initial peak amounts of the drug. Such barbiturates owe their extremely short duration of action to this phenomenon of rapid redistribution.

253-257. The answers are: 253-A, 254-D, 255-B, 256-C, 257-E. *(Gilman, ed 6. pp 353, 406, 546-548, 550-551, 556-557.)* The descriptions of the euphoric effects of cocaine are very similar to those attributed to amphetamines. Withdrawal of chronic cocaine administration results in depression, fatigue, prolonged sleep, hyperphagia and craving. Although some tolerance to the convulsant and cardiorespiratory effects of cocaine has been noted, the accepted view is that repeated use of cocaine may result in increased CNS sensitivity to the drug.

Heroin and other opioids exhibit a high degree of craving, tolerance, and physical dependence. The magnitude or rate of tolerance to all of the effects of opioids are not necessarily the same. The physical dependence is quite clear from the character and severity of withdrawal symptoms which include vomiting, spasms, abdominal cramps, diarrhea, and acid-base imbalances among others.

Tolerance to the anorectic, euphorigenic, hyperthermic, and lethal actions of amphetamines has been observed. This clearly results in the use of increased dosages to produce the desired effects. Abrupt cessation of amphetamine use does not cause major, observable physiological disruption.

Secobarbital exhibits the same pharmacological properties as other members of the barbiturate class. While there may be considerable tolerance to the sedative and intoxicating effects of the drug, the lethal dose is not much greater in addicted than in normal individuals. Severe withdrawal symptoms in epileptic patients may include grand mal seizures and delirium.

No current evidence exists that chlorpromazine, an antipsychotic agent, is addicting. Although some tolerance and physical dependence has been suggested, the failure to detect any EEG changes upon abrupt cessation of the drug implies that these effects are not of major importance. Chlorpromazine has a high therapeutic index and is a very safe drug.

Autonomic Nervous System

DIRECTIONS: Each question below contains five suggested answers. Choose the **one best** response to each question.

258. The drug of choice for the treatment of anaphylactic shock is

(A) histamine
(B) epinephrine
(C) norepinephrine
(D) isoproterenol
(E) diphenhydramine

259. Phenoxybenzamine (Dibenzyline) often causes an increase in heart rate and in the force of contraction by which of the following mechanisms?

(A) Stimulating cardiac β_1 receptors
(B) Antagonizing the vagal transmitter
(C) Releasing histamine from mast cells, which stimulates the heart
(D) Blocking peripheral vasoconstriction, which produces reflex stimulation of the heart
(E) Increasing the amount of calcium available to the heart

260. Which of the following statements about ergotamine in the treatment of migraine headaches is true?

(A) It has vasoconstrictive properties that may account for its efficacy
(B) It has adrenergic blocking properties that are responsible for its therapeutic benefit
(C) It will successfully terminate a migraine headache already in progress
(D) It is effective for the prevention of further migraine attacks
(E) It is easily tolerated when taken orally

261. The structure shown below is the prototype for which of the following classes of drugs?

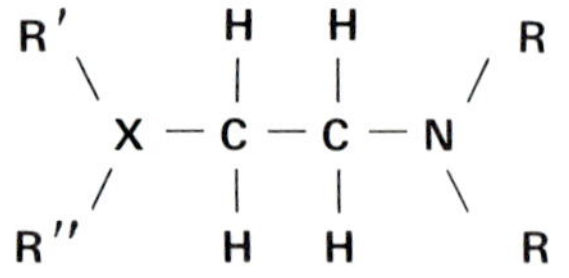

(A) Sympathomimetics
(B) Anticholinergics
(C) Local anesthetics
(D) Antihistaminics
(E) Antibiotics

262. A selective blockade of β-adrenergic receptors is produced by which of the following drugs?

(A) Guanethidine (Ismelin)
(B) Propranolol (Inderal)
(C) Scopolamine
(D) Nicotine
(E) Phentolamine (Regitine)

263. A 24-year-old man is brought to the emergency room by a group of friends who said that he had suddenly become restless, confused, and uncoordinated after taking some pills. Physical examination reveals increased body temperature, tachycardia, cutaneous flush, and widely dilated pupils unresponsive to light. The patient complains of dryness of the mouth. He probably ingested which of the following drugs?

(A) Codeine
(B) Aspirin
(C) Secobarbital
(D) Belladonna extract
(E) Chlordiazepoxide (Librium)

264. Functionally, a patient with myasthenia gravis resembles a person who has been treated with low doses of

(A) atropine
(B) tubocurarine
(C) methacholine
(D) muscarine
(E) propranolol (Inderal)

265. A selective cholinomimetic effect on the gastrointestinal and urinary tracts is produced by which of the following drugs?

(A) Methacholine
(B) Carbachol
(C) Bethanechol
(D) Neostigmine
(E) Edrophonium (Tensilon)

266. Cimetidine (Tagamet) is effective in treating duodenal ulcer because it

(A) strengthens the protective coating on the intestinal wall
(B) reduces parasympathetic-induced gastrointestinal secretions by competing at muscarinic receptors
(C) is an agonist at H_1 receptors and therefore reduces pepsin secretion
(D) blocks histamine stimulation of gastric acid secretion by H_2 receptors
(E) increases bicarbonate ion secretion, neutralizing the pH

267. All the following neurotransmitter receptor sites are β-adrenergic receptors EXCEPT for

(A) the ciliary muscle of the iris
(B) the radial muscle of the iris
(C) bronchial muscle
(D) the atrioventricular node
(E) the sinoatrial node

268. Phenylethanolamine-*N*-methyltransferase catalyzes the methylation of which of the following substances?

(A) Epinephrine
(B) Norepinephrine
(C) Serotonin
(D) Histidine
(E) Dihydroxyphenylalanine

269. The adrenal medulla secretes epinephrine in response to administration of

(A) atropine
(B) tubocurarine
(C) succinylcholine
(D) methyldopa (Aldomet)
(E) nicotine

270. In certain patients, the duration of apnea produced after administration of succinylcholine is hours rather than a few minutes. These patients probably have a deficiency of

(A) liver transglucosylase
(B) liver hydroxymethylase
(C) plasma cholinesterase
(D) plasma glycine transamidinase
(E) red blood cell glucose 6-phosphate dehydrogenase

271. A drug that acts effectively not only on α- but also on β_1- and β_2-adrenergic receptors is

(A) epinephrine
(B) norepinephrine
(C) isoproterenol
(D) phentolamine (Regitine)
(E) propranolol (Inderal)

272. All the following statements apply to succinylcholine EXCEPT that

(A) neuromuscular blockade may be enhanced in patients receiving streptomycin
(B) histamine release is stimulated
(C) muscular fasciculations occur briefly after administration
(D) muscles usually remain relaxed for one hour after intravenous infusion
(E) hexafluorenium bromide prolongs its effects

273. Norepinephrine, after having interacted with the receptor of the effector cell, is subject to inactivation by

(A) aromatic L-amino acid decarboxylase
(B) catechol-*O*-methyltransferase
(C) phenylethanolamine-*N*-methyltransferase
(D) dopamine β-hydroxylase
(E) tyrosine hydroxylase

274. Serotonin, a central nervous system transmitter, is found in the highest concentrations in which of the following areas of the brain?

(A) Thalamus
(B) Hypothalamus
(C) Cerebral cortex
(D) Basal ganglia
(E) Cerebral white matter

275. Phenylephrine is included in cold remedies sold over the counter because it

(A) causes vasoconstriction by alpha receptor stimulation
(B) prevents vasodilation by blocking beta receptors
(C) stimulates the central nervous system to increase blood flow
(D) reduces secretion by inhibiting parasympathetic stimulation
(E) is an antihistamine that reduces secretion

276. Ganglionic blocking drugs cause all the following effects EXCEPT

(A) vasodilatation
(B) decreased cardiac output
(C) mydriasis
(D) salivation
(E) decreased intestinal motility

277. A predictably dangerous side effect of propranolol (Inderal), which constitutes a contraindication to its clinical use in susceptible patients, is the induction of

(A) hypertension
(B) cardiac arrhythmia
(C) asthmatic attacks
(D) respiratory depression
(E) hypersensitivity

278. Metabolites of norepinephrine include all the following EXCEPT

(A) metanephrine
(B) normetanephrine
(C) 3,4-dihydroxymandelic acid
(D) 3-methoxy-4-hydroxymandelic acid
(E) 3-methoxy-4-hydroxyphenylglycol

279. The preferred drug for confirming the presence of pheochromocytoma in a patient who is severely hypertensive is

(A) piperoxan
(B) phenoxybenzamine (Dibenzyline)
(C) histamine
(D) phentolamine (Regitine)
(E) methacholine

280. The mechanism of action of the long-lasting organic phosphate anticholinesterases is

(A) splitting of polypeptide bonds in cholinesterases
(B) phosphorylation of the anionic site of cholinesterases
(C) phosphorylation of the esteratic site of cholinesterases
(D) acetylation of the anionic site of cholinesterases
(E) acetylation of the esteratic site of cholinesterases

DIRECTIONS: Each question below contains four suggested answers of which **one** or **more** is correct. Choose the answer:

A	if	**1, 2, and 3**	are correct
B	if	**1 and 3**	are correct
C	if	**2 and 4**	are correct
D	if	**4**	is correct
E	if	**1, 2, 3, and 4**	are correct

281. The biochemical actions of methyldopa (Aldomet) include which of the following?

(1) Inhibition of amino acid decarboxylase
(2) Inhibition of tyrosine hydroxylase
(3) Interruption of serotonin synthesis
(4) Interruption of steroid synthesis

282. Presynaptic α receptors are blocked by which of the following drugs?

(1) Phenoxybenzamine (Dibenzyline)
A (2) Phentolamine (Regitine)
(3) Tolazoline (Priscoline)
(4) Prazosin (Minipress)

283. Poisoning by an organophosphate insecticide causes which of the following clinical findings?

(1) Increased bronchial secretions
(2) Constipation
B (3) Miosis
(4) Tetanus

284. Bronchodilation can be produced by administration of

(1) theophylline
(2) aminophylline
(3) isoproterenol
(4) phenoxybenzamine (Dibenzyline)

285. Carbachol and bethanechol have pharmacokinetic properties that include

(1) vasodilation and negative chronotropic and inotropic effects
(2) virtually total resistance to hydrolysis by either acetylcholinesterase or nonspecific cholinesterase
(3) muscarinic activity that is not blocked by atropine
(4) relatively selective action on the smooth muscle of the gastrointestinal tract and urinary bladder

286. Administration of intravenous epinephrine would cause which of the following physiologic changes?

(1) Increase in coronary blood flow
B (2) Decrease in both systolic and diastolic pressures by approximately 10 mm Hg
(3) Reduction in cutaneous blood flow
(4) Decrease in arterial and venous pulmonary pressures

287. Dopamine is used in the treatment of cardiogenic shock and septic shock because it

(1) increases cardiac output
(2) prevents the release of protease-activating factors
(3) dilates renal blood vessels
(4) increases activity of the corpus striatum

288. Quaternary ammonium ganglionic blocking agents have the ability to

(1) act by preventing depolarizing actions of acetylcholine or by producing persistent depolarization
(2) be excreted by the liver
(3) produce orthostatic hypotension
(4) be pharmacologically effective in oral preparations

289. The symptoms of patients who have myasthenia gravis may be transiently improved by treatment with

(1) neostigmine (Prostigmin)
(2) tubocurarine chloride
(3) edrophonium (Tensilon)
(4) atropine

290. Methylation can inactivate which of the following neurotransmitters?

(1) Epinephrine
(2) Norepinephrine
(3) Histamine
(4) 5-Hydroxytryptamine

291. Drugs that contain a quaternary amino group and are, therefore, less able to cross biologic membranes include

(1) physostigmine (Antilirium)
(2) neostigmine (Prostigmin)
(3) epinephrine
(4) acetylcholine

292. Atropine blocks the effect of acetylcholine at which of the following sites?

(1) Exocrine glands
(2) Cardiac muscle
(3) Smooth muscle
(4) Skeletal muscle

293. The combination of β-adrenergic stimulation and α-adrenergic blockade causes

(1) uterine relaxation
(2) bronchodilation
(3) vasodilation
(4) mydriasis

294. Urinary 5-hydroxyindoleacetic acid excretion may be greatly increased in which of the following circumstances?

(1) In the presence of carcinoid tumor
(2) After ingestion of bananas
(3) After administration of reserpine
(4) After administration of monoamine oxidase inhibitors

SUMMARY OF DIRECTIONS

A	B	C	D	E
1, 2, 3 only	1, 3 only	2, 4 only	4 only	All are correct

295. Neostigmine (Prostigmin) differs from physostigmine (Antilirium) because neostigmine

(1) has an additional direct effect at neuromuscular junctions
(2) is less well absorbed from the gastrointestinal tract
(3) is a quaternary ammonium compound, and physostigmine is a tertiary amine
(4) is a reversible cholinesterase inhibitor, whereas physostigmine is an irreversible one

296. Epinephrine is added to local anesthetics in order to

(1) stimulate local wound repair
(2) promote hemostasis
(3) facilitate their dissemination along nerves and fascial planes
(4) retard their absorption

297. Catecholamines cause hyperglycemia through which of the following mechanisms?

(1) Inhibition of insulin release
(2) Inhibition of hepatic glycogen synthase
(3) Stimulation of glycogen phosphorylase
(4) Direct inhibition of glucose transport systems

DIRECTIONS: The groups of questions below consist of lettered choices followed by several numbered items. For each numbered item select the **one** lettered choice with which it is **most** closely associated. Each lettered choice may be used once, more than once, or not at all.

Questions 298-302

For each pharmacologic action listed, select the drug with which it is most likely to be associated.

(A) Pralidoxime (Protopam)
(B) Prazosin (Minipress)
(C) Scopolamine
(D) Timolol (Timoptic)
(E) Phenoxybenzamine (Dibenzyline)

298. Reduces intraocular pressure

299. Counters toxic effects of organophosphates

300. Blocks muscarinic sites in the periphery and central nervous system

301. Reacts irreversibly with receptors

302. Decreases heart rate, especially when sympathetic activity is high

Questions 303-307

For each of the following drugs, select the enzyme that it inhibits.

(A) Carbonic anhydrase
(B) Cholinesterase
(C) Monoamine oxidase
(D) Phosphodiesterase
(E) Xanthine oxidase

303. Acetazolamide

304. Allopurinol

305. Theophylline

306. Pyridostigmine

307. Tranylcypromine

Questions 308-310

For each anatomic site listed, select the catecholamine neurotransmitter with which it is most likely to be associated.

(A) Dopamine
(B) Serotonin
(C) Epinephrine
(D) Norepinephrine
(E) Acetylcholine

308. Adrenergic fibers

309. Adrenal medulla

310. Caudate nucleus

Questions 311-313

For each of the following acetylcholine-sensitive receptors, select the most effective acetylcholine antagonist.

(A) Muscarine
(B) Tubocurarine
(C) Atropine
(D) Nicotine
(E) Hexamethonium

311. Cardiac muscle

312. Skeletal muscle

313. Ganglia

Questions 314-318

For each of the following naturally occurring amines, select the appropriate structure.

A
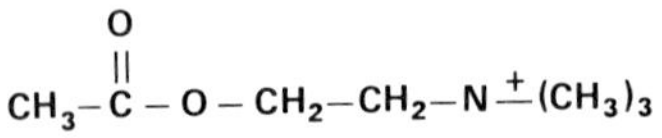

B
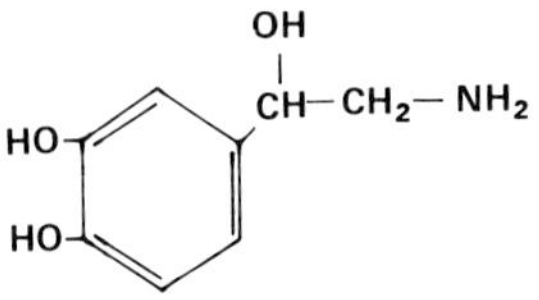

C
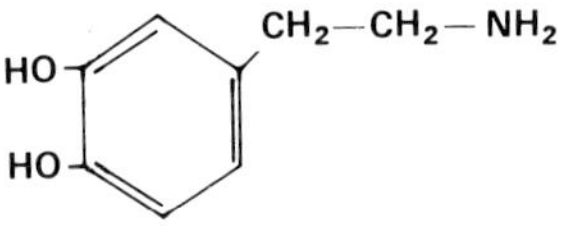

D
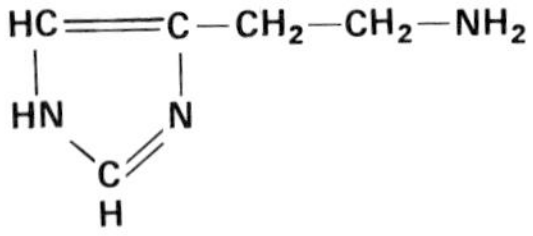

E
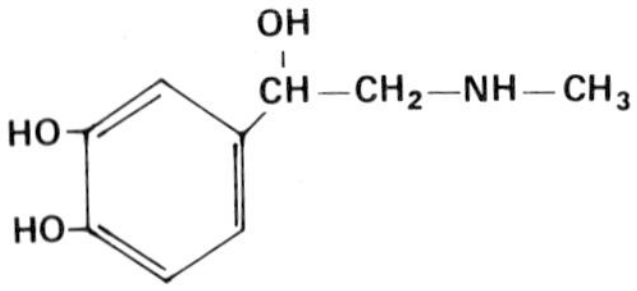

314. Acetylcholine
315. Dopamine
316. Norepinephrine
317. Histamine
318. Epinephrine

Questions 319-321

For each of the following neurotransmitters, select the amino acid from which it is synthesized.

(A) Tyrosine
(B) Serine
(C) Histidine
(D) Tryptophan
(E) Hydroxyproline

319. Epinephrine
320. Histamine
321. Serotonin

Questions 322-327

For each of the following drugs, select its appropriate site of action in the acetylcholine system shown below.

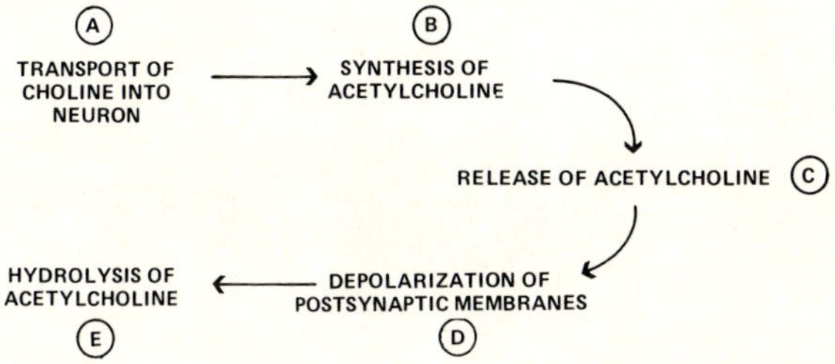

322. Botulinus toxin
323. Diisopropyl fluorophosphate
324. Tubocurarine
325. Hemicholinium
326. Hexamethonium
327. Pilocarpine

Questions 328-331

Match the following.

(A) Methysergide
(B) Methscopolamine
(C) Methacholine
(D) Methoxsalen (Oxsoralen)
(E) Methyldopa (Aldomet)

328. An antagonist of 5-hydroxytryptamine

329. Slowly hydrolyzed by acetylcholinesterase

330. Used in treatment of essential hypertension

331. A semisynthetic antagonist of muscarinic cholinergic receptors

Autonomic Nervous System

Answers

258. The answer is B. *(Gilman, ed 6. p 171.)* Epinephrine is the drug of choice to relieve the symptoms of an acute hypersensitivity reaction to allergens (anaphylactic shock). Subcutaneous administration rapidly relieves itching and urticaria and may save the life of the patient when laryngeal edema threatens suffocation. Angioedema is responsive to antihistaminics, but epinephrine is necessary in the event of a severe reaction.

259. The answer is D. *(Craig, p 146.)* Phenoxybenzamine is an inhibitor of both α_1 and α_2 receptors. It prevents vasoconstriction of peripheral blood vessels by endogenous catecholamines, an effect that is more pronounced when sympathetic activity is high. The resulting hypotension causes a reflex stimulation of the heart. Because this stimulation occurs through β receptors, it is not blocked by phenoxybenzamine.

260. The answer is A. *(Gilman, ed 6. pp 946-947.)* Ergotamine, by virtue of its vasoconstrictive properties rather than its adrenergic blocking action, is the drug of choice for combating an incipient attack of migraine headache; it has been used for this purpose since 1926. Although long-term treatment with this nonsedative, nonanalgesic drug does not decrease the frequency of or prevent the migraine attacks, administration of oral doses is recommended at the beginning of an attack, especially during the prodromal stage, despite the fact that ergotamine is poorly absorbed by the gastrointestinal mucosa and its effects are much slower than when given parenterally. (Administration before the prodromal stage may, in fact, cause an attack, perhaps by exacerbating the vasoconstriction that is thought to occur prior to this stage.) Oral ergotamine provides relief in five hours and is generally the preferred route for treatment of mild attacks. Administration of this most potent of the ergot alkaloids at the peak of a migraine episode requires effective doses larger than those administered during the prodromal stage and is associated with a delayed onset of action and with side effects such as nausea, vomiting, pruritus, and disturbances in heart rate.

261. The answer is D. *(Gilman, ed 6. p 623.)* The structure shown in the question is the general structural formula for most antihistaminic agents. The core of the structure consists of an ethylamine group ($-CH_2CH_2N=$) that is also found in histamine. Antihistamines with this structure are H_1-receptor antagonists. Histamine antagonists compete with agonist molecules for positions on the receptive sites of effector cells.

262. The answer is B. *(Gilman, ed 6. pp 190, 194.)* Propranolol (Inderal) is the prototype drug of the class that acts as a selective β-adrenergic blocker. This class of drugs slows the heart rate, decreases cardiac output, attenuates mechanical systole, and causes a slight lowering of blood pressure. β-Blockers are used clinically in the treatment of angina pectoris, hypertension, and arrhythmias such as supraventricular arrhythmias. Successful treatment of hyperthyroidism and associated cardiovascular disturbances with propranolol has been reported, but the use of the β-adrenergic blocking agent in hyperthyroidism on a long-term basis requires further evaluation. The drug has been noted to mask continuing hyperthyroidism.

263. The answer is D. *(Gilman, ed 6. p 127.)* The history and clinical findings in the patient presented in the question are indicative of widespread parasympathetic blockade. Symptoms and signs of such blockade should immediately arouse suspicion of belladonna poisoning. When belladonna poisoning is suspected but questionable, subcutaneous injection of 1 mg of physostigmine (Antilirium) can be diagnostic—if salivation, sweating, and intestinal hyperactivity do not occur following the injection, belladonna intoxication is almost certain.

264. The answer is B. *(Craig, pp 174, 206-207.)* A disturbance of neuromuscular transmission is the essential functional manifestation in both myasthenia gravis and in a patient who has received small doses of tubocurarine chloride. Tubocurarine is a nondepolarizing neuromuscular blocking agent that competes with acetylcholine for the receptor. In both situations, improvement may be achieved by administration of anticholinesterase inhibitors such as physostigmine, neostigmine, and edrophonium.

265. The answer is C. *(Craig, pp 160-161, 174-175.)* Bethanechol is the parasympathomimetic drug of choice for postoperative urinary distress and abdominal distension. Methacholine is used only as a diagnostic tool to detect poisoning due to belladonna alkaloids. Carbachol may be used in glaucoma; neostigmine and edrophonium (Tensilon) may be used, respectively, in the treatment and diagnosis of myasthenia gravis.

266. The answer is D. *(Gilman, ed 6. pp 630-631.)* Cimetidine (Tagamet) is a commonly prescribed histamine antagonist that is specific for H_2 receptors. Cimetidine prevents histamine-stimulated gastric acid secretion, gastrin-induced secretion, and acetylcholine-induced secretion. Placebo-treated duodenal ulcers heal in about 60-70 percent of affected patients in the United States; cimetidine-treated ulcers heal in 70-80 percent of patients.

267. The answer is B. *(Gilman, ed 6. p 60.)* The radial muscle of the iris contains α-adrenergic receptors; when exposed to such α-receptor agonists as phenylephrine, the muscle contracts, resulting in mydriasis. Miosis occurs when the ciliary muscle, which contains β receptors, relaxes. Bronchial muscle, the atrioventricular node, and the sinoatrial node are among other sites that contain β receptors.

268. The answer is B. *(Cooper, ed 4. p 137.)* Phenylethanolamine-*N*-methyltransferase catalyzes the methylation of the terminal amino group of norepinephrine, an action resulting in the formation of epinephrine. The addition of the methyl group, derived from the transmethylation donor *S*-adenosylmethionine, greatly increases the feeble β_2 activity of norepinephrine. This cytoplasmic enzyme is present largely in the adrenal medulla.

269. The answer is E. *(Craig, p 107.)* The adrenal medulla as a modified sympathetic ganglion responds to acetylcholine, which is the ganglionic mediator of both parasympathetic and sympathetic nerves. Nicotine mimics these cholinergic effects. Atropine, tubocurarine, and succinylcholine inhibit postsynaptic membrane depolarization. Methyldopa (Aldomet) inhibits the synthesis of epinephrine and norepinephrine.

270. The answer is C. *(Gilman, ed 6. p 230.)* Normal plasma cholinesterase enzymatically destroys succinylcholine and is responsible for its short duration of action. Succinylcholine-induced paralysis usually lasts for five minutes (during which time artificial respiration is needed). Individuals who are homozygous for a deficient plasma cholinesterase, therefore, remain paralyzed much longer than the average person following the administration of succinylcholine. In rare instances, some individuals completely lack plasma cholinesterase.

271. The answer is A. *(Gilman, ed 6. p 139.)* Norepinephrine, epinephrine, and isoproterenol are clinically important, chemically related drugs that exert prominent actions on adrenergic receptors. The structure of norepinephrine is:

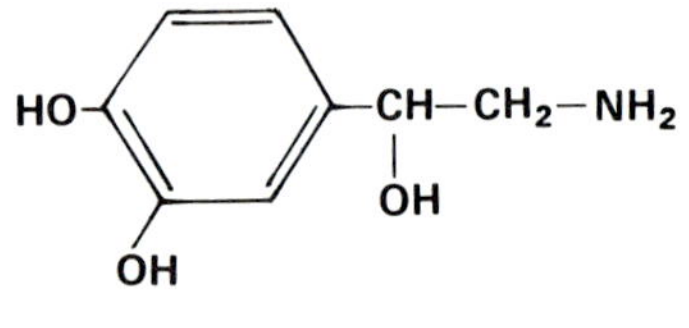

It has stronger effects on α- than β-adrenergic receptors; epinephrine, which has a methyl group on the terminal nitrogen, has marked effects on α, β_1, and β_2 receptors. Isoproterenol, which has an isopropyl substituent on the amino group, has effects limited largely to the two β receptors. The size of the alkyl substituent on the terminal amino group is associated with the intensity of the effects on α and β receptors: in general, as the size of the substituent increases, the action on α receptors decreases and on β receptors increases. Phentolamine (Regitine) and propranolol (Inderal) are chemically dissimilar: the former has the ability to block α receptors, whereas the latter blocks both β receptors.

272. **The answer is D.** *(Gilman, ed 6. pp 225-231.)* Succinylcholine is a depolarizing neuromuscular blocking agent used for producing muscle relaxation during surgery. When given intravenously, there are brief muscle fasciculations followed by relaxation within 1 or 2 minutes. Succinylcholine is rapidly cleaved by a pseudocholinesterase, thus its effect does not last more than 5 minutes unless hydrolysis is prevented by hexafluorenium bromide, a pseudocholinesterase inhibitor. Succinylcholine stimulates histamine release, although not as much as tubocurarine. Streptomycin at high concentrations can cause neuromuscular blockade and may be synergistic with succinylcholine.

273. **The answer is B.** *(Gilman, ed 6. p 77.)* Catechol-*O*-methyltransferase inactivates norepinephrine by methylation to normetanephrine. Tyrosine hydroxylase is the rate-limiting enzyme of catecholamine synthesis; dopamine β hydroxylase and aromatic L-amino acid decarboxylase are also involved in synthesis. Phenylethanolamine-*N*-methyl-transferase is a catalyst in the formation of epinephrine from norepinephrine.

274. **The answer is B.** *(Craig, pp 389-391.)* Approximately 2 percent of the total serotonin in the mammalian body is located within the central nervous system, especially in the pineal gland and hypothalamus. The enterochromaffin cells of the intestine contain about 90 percent of this endogenously produced amine chemically known as 5-hydroxytryptamine (5-HT). Independent discoveries of 5-HT in serum and in the enterochromaffin cells resulted in the naming of the amine as serotonin and enteramine. Many studies have been conducted on the role of 5-HT in mood, behavioral, and various mental disorders and in the motility of the intestine.

275. **The answer is A.** *(Gilman, ed 6. pp 165, 168.)* Phenylephrine stimulates postsynaptic α receptors but has little effect on β receptors. When applied directly to nasal mucosal tissue, it causes vasoconstriction, which reduces congestion. Phenylephrine is sometimes included in oral preparations, but a dose high enough to be effective as a nasal decongestant would produce generalized vasoconstriction and hypertension.

276. The answer is D. *(Gilman, ed 6. p 216.)* The alterations caused by ganglionic blocking agents in physiologic processes can be predicted by a knowledge of which divisions of the autonomic nervous system exert dominant control over various organs. Adrenergic blockade results in arteriolar vasodilatation and decreased cardiac output, which is probably secondary to decreased venous return. In addition, generalized ganglionic blockade may also result in bladder and gastrointestinal atony, xerostomia, decreased perspiration, and mydriasis.

277. The answer is C. *(Gilman, ed 6. pp 193-194.)* The chief danger of therapy with β-adrenergic blocking agents such as propranolol (Inderal) is associated with the blockade itself. β-Adrenergic blockade results in an increase in airway resistance that can be fatal in asthmatic patients. Hypersensitivity reactions such as rash, fever, and purpura are rare and necessitate discontinuation of therapy.

278. The answer is A. *(Gilman, ed 6. pp 76-77.)* Metanephrine is a metabolite in the metabolic pathway of epinephrine. By the action of monoamine oxidase (MAO), norepinephrine can be oxidatively deaminated to 3,4-dihydroxymandelic acid; by the action of catechol-*O*-methyltransferase (COMT), it can be methylated to normetanephrine. The major excretory product of catecholamine metabolism is 3-methoxy-4-hydroxymandelic acid (also known as vanillylmandelic acid [VMA], a generally established misnomer). It is the product of the action of COMT on 3,4-dihydroxymandelic acid and of the action of MAO on metanephrine and normetanephrine. Although widely distributed in the human body and present in the highest concentration in the liver and kidney, MAO catalyzes the reduction—mostly in the central nervous system—of some of the oxidation products of normetanephrine and metanephrine to 3-methoxy-4-hydroxyphenylglycol.

279. The answer is D. *(Gilman, ed 6. p 186.)* Phentolamine mesylate, U.S.P., (Regitine) may be administered intravenously or intramuscularly to hypertensive patients in whom the diagnosis of pheochromocytoma is suspected. A positive test for this pharmacologic method of diagnosing pheochromocytoma consists of decreases of systolic and diastolic pressures of 35 and 25 mm Hg, respectively, within about 2 minutes after intravenous injection or within about 20 minutes after intramuscular injection. The diagnosis of pheochromocytoma is not excluded by a negative test result, especially for patients who have paroxysmal hypertension. The use of a drug that has hypotensive effects is preferred in the pharmacologic diagnosis of pheochromocytoma, a tumor whose cardinal symptom is hypertension and exacerbation of which may result in death. An increase in blood pressure is the usual consequence of the administration of histamine or methacholine in persons who have pheochromocytoma. According to current studies, the use of phentolamine in screening tests for hypertension has been supplanted by assays of urinary levels of catecholamines and other substances; phentolamine is now recommended as a diagnostic pharmacologic agent in providing confirmation of other evidence of pheochromocytoma.

280. The answer is C. *(Craig, pp 170-172.)* During the hydrolysis of acetylcholine by acetylcholinesterase, the enzyme binds to the substrate by virtue of the electrostatic attraction between the anionic site of the enzyme and the quaternary nitrogen of acetylcholine. In addition, the electrophilic carbon of the carbonyl group of acetylcholine interacts with the nearby nucleophilic esteratic site of the enzyme. As a result of this attraction and interaction, a complex is formed and subsequently cleaved to yield the products choline and the acetylated enzyme. Hydrolysis then rapidly yields acetic acid and the regenerated active enzyme. Those organophosphorus compounds that inhibit cholinesterase activity react with the esteratic site in a manner similar to the processes that occur in the hydrolysis of acetylcholine but phosphorylate rather than acetylate the enzyme. The phosphorylated enzyme does not readily undergo hydrolysis, and thus the enzyme is inactivated.

281. The answer is B (1, 3). *(Gilman, ed 6. p 794.)* Methyldopa (Aldomet) is an effective inhibitor of L-aromatic amino acid decarboxylase, which in turn inhibits decarboxylation of both dopa and serotonin. Methyldopa is metabolized to α-methylnorepinephrine, which may act as a "false transmitter." The hypotensive effect of methyldopa is considered to be due to its metabolite rather than to its enzyme inhibition activity.

282. The answer is A (1, 2, 3). *(Craig, pp 143-144.)* Phenoxybenzamine, phentolamine, tolazoline, and prazosin all are α-adrenergic antagonists. Only prazosin is specific for α_1-postsynaptic receptors. α_2 Receptors, which are located on nerve terminals, when activated cause a reduction in further release of norepinephrine. Therefore, although phenoxybenzamine, phentolamine, and tolazoline block stimulation by competing with norepinephrine at postsynaptic receptors, they also cause more norepinephrine to be released by blocking presynaptic receptors.

283. The answer is B (1, 3). *(Gilman, ed 6. pp 101-110.)* Organophosphates combine covalently with cholinesterases, preventing the hydrolysis of acetylcholine. Excess acetylcholine stimulates organs and ganglia that have receptors. Therefore, glands innervated by postganglionic cholinergic fibers are stimulated, and secretions from bronchial, sweat, and salivary glands increase. Acetylcholine increases activity of the gastrointestinal tract and gastric acid secretion. Acetylcholine also contracts the sphincter muscle of the iris, causing miosis. Initially, acetylcholine may cause contractions of skeletal muscles, but continued exposure to the agent causes depolarization blockade resulting in fasciculations and weakness.

284. The answer is A (1, 2, 3). *(Craig, pp 129, 470.)* Isoproterenol, as a potent activator of β receptors, produces bronchodilatation. Several drugs such as ephedrine and some theophylline derivatives are also used as bronchodilators. Phenoxybenzamine (Dibenzyline) is an α-adrenergic blocking agent but exerts no direct effect on β-adrenergic receptors.

285. The answer is C (2, 4). *(Gilman, ed 6. pp 92-94.)* Compared to acetylcholine, the cardiovascular effects of carbachol and bethanechol are inconspicuous. These two drugs resist hydrolysis by acetylcholinesterase and nonspecific esterase. Also in contrast to acetylcholine, they selectively stimulate the urinary, as well as the gastrointestinal, tract. The muscarinic effects of all the parasympathomimetic drugs are blocked by atropine.

286. The answer is B (1, 3). *(Gilman, ed 6. pp 144-146.)* Epinephrine is one of the most potent vasopressor drugs. Given intravenously, it increases systolic pressure more than diastolic pressure. Cutaneous blood flow is significantly reduced, but coronary blood flow is enhanced, owing chiefly to a metabolic dilator effect associated with stronger myocardial contraction and the influence of local metabolites produced by a relatively hypoxic myocardium. Pulmonary venous pressure increases secondary to an increase in left atrial pressure.

287. The answer is B (1, 3). *(Craig, p 132.)* Damage associated with shock is caused by inadequate circulation—tissues are inadequately perfused and toxic compounds accumulate in the blood. Dopamine increases blood flow by stimulating β receptors in the heart, which increase the strength of myocardial contraction. Dopamine does not cause vasodilation of peripheral blood vessels, but does dilate blood vessels in the kidney through specific dopaminergic receptors. Increased blood flow in the kidney may reduce the accumulation of toxic substances.

288. The answer is B (1, 3). *(Craig, pp 198-199.)* Ganglionic blocking agents such as hexamethonium are used mainly for decreasing the influence on the circulatory system of the sympathetic branch of the autonomic nervous system. They tend to lower blood pressure by decreasing sympathetic vascular tone, which prevents compensatory vasoconstriction in response to postural changes. Ganglionic blocking agents are poorly absorbed from the gastrointestinal tract and are excreted via the kidney.

289. The answer is B (1, 3). *(Gilman, ed 6. pp 114-116.)* Administration of the anticholinesterases neostigmine (Prostigmin) and edrophonium (Tensilon) has been used to improve the symptoms of patients who have myasthenia gravis. Neostigmine (in oral doses for prolonged symptomatic management in the absence of dysphagia, or in parenteral doses for the acute crisis) is generally considered the drug of choice to improve muscle strength of affected patients. Although both agents can be used in the differential diagnosis of myasthenia gravis, edrophonium is usually recommended as the preferred diagnostic agent due to its more rapid onset and brief duration of physiologic action, according to the results of recent studies. Tubocurarine exacerbates the symptoms of myasthenia gravis.

290. The answer is A (1, 2, 3). *(Gilman, ed 6. pp 77, 618, 637.)* Methylation of norepinephrine yields the equally potent transmitter epinephrine. However, both epinephrine and norepinephrine may be inactivated by methylation to metanephrine and normetanephrine, respectively. Histamine is also inactivated by methylation. Serotonin (5-hydroxytryptamine) is inactivated by oxidation to 5-hydroxyindoleacetic acid.

291. The answer is C (2, 4). *(Gilman, ed 6. pp 102, 104.)* Neostigmine (Prostigmin) and acetylcholine both contain quaternary ammonium groups. As a result, neostigmine is absorbed from the gastrointestinal tract more slowly than physostigmine (Antilirium), a related anticholinesterase with tertiary amino groups. Epinephrine has a secondary amino group.

292. The answer is A (1, 2, 3). *(Craig, pp 108-109.)* Atropine blocks the effect of acetylcholine on smooth and cardiac muscles and on exocrine glands. It does not block the effect of acetylcholine on skeletal muscle or ganglia. Tubocurarine inhibits the skeletal neuromuscular action of acetylcholine with essentially no effect on smooth muscle.

293. The answer is A (1, 2, 3). *(Gilman, ed 6. pp 60-61.)* β-Adrenergic receptor stimulation concomitant with α-adrenergic receptor blockade would cause effects characteristic of the activation of both β_1- and β_2-adrenergic receptors. The β_1-mediated effects would include myocardial stimulation and relaxation of the gastrointestinal tract; β_2-mediated effects would include bronchodilation, vasodilation, and relaxation of the uterus.

294. The answer is A (1, 2, 3). *(Gilman, ed 6. pp 633, 636-638.)* The daily urinary output (3 to 10 mg for a normal adult) of 5-hydroxyindoleacetic acid, a catabolic metabolite of serotonin (5-hydroxytryptamine), is markedly increased when a carcinoid tumor is present, after ingestion of bananas (which contain a high quantity of serotonin), and after administration of reserpine. The latter substance promotes the release of serotonin from its binding sites. In the mammalian body, the synthesis of serotonin from tryptophan occurs predominantly in the enterochromaffin cells of the intestine, a small percentage is synthesized in the central nervous system, and about 8 percent is stored rather than synthesized in the platelets. Because monoamine oxidase (MAO) catalyzes the biotransformation of serotonin to 5-hydroxyindoleacetic acid, administration of MAO inhibitors results in decreased production of the end product.

295. The answer is A (1, 2, 3). *(Gilman, ed 6. pp 104, 107-108.)* Neostigmine is a quaternary ammonium compound, whereas physostigmine is a tertiary amine, as shown by the structural formulas:

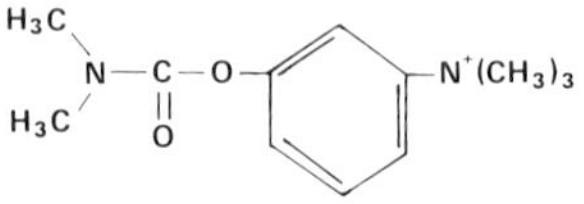

Neostigmine

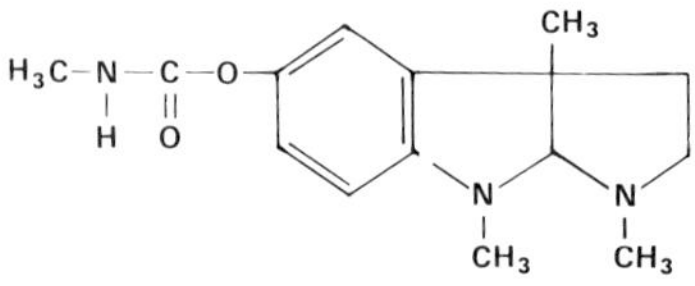

Physostigmine

Neostigmine, parenterally administered, will act directly at the neuromuscular junction—even in the absence of cholinesterase activity—and some of its effects are attributable to its anticholinesterase action. Although gastrointestinal absorption of both compounds is variable, neostigmine is absorbed less efficiently than physostigmine. Both drugs are reversible anticholinesterases.

296. The answer is D (4). *(Gilman, ed 6. pp 304, 308.)* The addition of vasoconstrictors, such as epinephrine, to local anesthetic preparations is a common practice in order to prevent their rapid absorption, to prolong the local action, and to decrease the systemic reaction. The vasoconstrictor-anesthetic ratio ranges from 1:100,000 to 1:500,000. Lidocaine (Xylocaine), compared to procaine (Novocaine), is more potent, has a shorter period for its onset of action, and has a duration of action twice as long. The duration of action for infiltration anesthesia of procaine and lidocaine is greatly increased by the addition of epinephrine.

297. The answer is A (1, 2, 3). *(Gilman, ed 6. pp 78-79.)* Catecholamines exert several metabolic effects, including hyperglycemia and hyperlipemia. Hyperglycemia is caused by inhibition of glycogen synthase, which uses glucose to make glycogen, and by stimulation of glycogen phosphorylase, which converts glycogen back to glucose. In addition, although β-receptor stimulation releases insulin, the predominant effect of catecholamines is to inhibit insulin release through α receptors.

298-302. The answers are: 298-D, 299-A, 300-C, 301-E, 302-D. *(Craig, pp 145-146, 151-154, 170, 176, 180-184.)* Timolol is a β-receptor antagonist. It does not show specificity for β_1 or β_2 receptors and, therefore, decreases the heart rate by blocking the action of endogenous catecholamines. Timolol, used to lower intraocular pressure in patients with chronic open-angle glaucoma, presumably by decreasing production of aqueous humor, is more effective than other drugs in the treatment of glaucoma.

Organophosphates react with acetylcholinesterase to phosphorylate the enzyme, thus rendering it inactive, inasmuch as the phosphoenzyme hydrolyzes very slowly. Pralidoxime is an oxime that can cause dephosphorylation of the enzyme if it is administered within a few hours after the organophosphates. If not administered promptly, the phosphoenzyme will lose an alkoxy group and then cannot be dephosphorylated. Pralidoxime is positively charged and, although unable to enter the central nervous system, it does decrease blockade at the neuromuscular junction.

Scopolamine is a muscarinic blocking agent that easily crosses the blood-brain barrier. The blocking of muscarinic receptors causes cycloplegia, decreased secretions in the gastrointestinal tract and in the lung, urinary retention, and bronchial dilation. Because of its inhibitory effects on secretion, scopolamine is found in many over-the-counter cold medications.

Phenoxybenzamine is a haloalkylamine related to the nitrogen mustards. It reacts covalently with receptors to produce an irreversible blockade and, therefore, is long-acting. Phenoxybenzamine is primarily an α-adrenergic inhibitor at clinical doses but can also antagonize histamine. At higher doses, it can antagonize responses to acetylcholine and serotonin.

Prazosin is a reversible blocker of postsynaptic α receptors, unlike phenoxybenzamine, which reacts at both pre- and postsynaptic receptors. Prazosin is used to treat hypertension, whereas nonspecific α blockers are not, because prazosin does not block feedback at the presynaptic terminals. When feedback is blocked by nonspecific antagonists, the resulting increase in secretion of catecholamines allows them to compete with reversible antagonists.

303-307. The answers are: 303-A, 304-E, 305-D, 306-B, 307-C. *(Craig, pp 168, 329, 523, 935, 939-940.)* Acetazolamide is administered as a diuretic, as an anticonvulsant, and in the treatment of glaucoma, in which it acts to reduce the rate of formation of aqueous humor. All three actions generally are attributed to the ability of this nonbacteriostatic sulfonamide to inhibit the enzyme carbonic anhydrase.

Allopurinol inhibits xanthine oxidase, the enzyme primarily responsible for the oxidation of hypoxanthine and xanthine to uric acid. In patients who have gout and in whom hyperuricemia leads to the deposition of urates in joints and in tissues, allopurinol-induced inhibition of xanthine oxidase lowers circulating levels of uric acid to concentrations below the saturation point, thus suppressing the precipitation of urates. Allopurinol also prevents the synthesis of purines by depleting 5′-phosphoribosylpyrophosphate.

Theophylline, a methylated xanthine that has bronchodilating, diuretic, and cardiac-stimulant properties, is an inhibitor of phosphodiesterase, the enzyme responsible for the destruction of cyclic AMP. The actions of theophylline are thought to be the result of accumulation of cyclic AMP. Theophylline is used mainly to treat asthma.

Pyridostigmine is a "reversible" inhibitor of the cholinesterases. The structure of pyridostigmine includes a dimethylcarbamate side chain and a quaternary nitrogen atom within the ring. These moieties account for the pharmacologic properties of pyridostigmine and other related drugs, such as neostigmine.

Tranylcypromine is an antidepressant drug and an inhibitor of monoamine oxidase. Its antidepressant effect probably is due to the accumulation of norepinephrine in the brain as a consequence of inhibition of the enzyme. The other two monoamine oxidase inhibitors currently used are the hydrazide derivatives isocarboxazid and phenelzine.

308-310. The answers are: 308-D, 309-C, 310-A. *(Cooper, ed 4. pp 125-127, 175-179.)* Dopamine is formed from tyrosine by hydroxylation with tyrosine hydroxylase and the removal of a CO_2 group by aromatic amino acid decarboxylase. The catecholamine is found in high concentrations in parts of the brain: the caudate nucleus, the median eminence, the tuberculum olfactorium, and the nucleus accumbens. Dopamine appears to act as an inhibitory neurotransmitter.

Norepinephrine is synthesized from dopamine by dopamine-β-oxidase, which hydroxylates the β carbon. This enzyme is localized in the amine storage granules. Norepinephrine is found in adrenergic fibers, the adrenal medulla, and in neurons in the locus ceruleus and lateral ventral tegmental fields of the central nervous system.

Epinephrine is synthesized from norepinephrine in the adrenal medulla. Norepinephrine is methylated by phenylethanolamine-*N*-methyltransferase. Neurons containing this enzyme are also found in the central nervous system.

311-313. The answers are: 311-C, 312-B, 313-E. *(Gilman, ed 6. pp 83-84.)* Atropine is a competitive antagonist of acetylcholine. It binds to muscarinic receptors, which are found on cardiac muscle, smooth muscle, gland cells innervated by parasympathetic fibers, and in the central nervous system.

The receptors for acetylcholine on skeletal muscle are nicotinic. Atropine does not affect action of acetylcholine at these sites, but the effects are blocked by *d*-tubocurarine. Tubocurarine can also affect ganglionic nicotinic sites, although it is more effective at the neuromuscular junction.

Neurons in the ganglia of both the parasympathetic and the sympathetic nervous system have nicotinic receptors for acetylcholine. The action of acetylcholine at both these sites can be inhibited by hexamethonium. The length of the carbon chain, 6 carbons, is necessary for the ganglionic specificity of hexamethonium.

314-318. The answers are: 314-A, 315-C, 316-B, 317-D, 318-E. *(Cooper, ed 4. pp 78, 130-131, 354.)* Acetylcholine, which serves as the neurotransmitter at some synapses within the central nervous system, at autonomic ganglia, and at many peripheral neuroeffector sites, is an ester formed within the cholinergic neuron by the acetylation of choline. The acetylation reaction is catalyzed by the enzyme choline acetyltransferase (choline acetylase). After its release, acetylcholine is usually rapidly hydrolyzed by the enzyme acetylcholinesterase.

Dopamine is the neurotransmitter at selected synapses within the central nervous system and probably within some autonomic ganglia. It is formed within the neuron by the ring hydroxylation of phenylalanine and the subsequent decarboxylation of the resultant dihydroxyphenylalanine. Routes of metabolism of neuronally released dopamine include oxidation by monoamine oxidase and aldehyde dehydrogenase to 3,4-dihydroxyphenylacetic acid and methylation by catechol-*O*-methyltransferase to 3-methoxydopamine.

Norepinephrine is the principal neurotransmitter at peripheral autonomic adrenergic neuroeffector junctions, is synthesized within the adrenergic neuron by the β-hydroxylation of dopamine, and—in contrast to epinephrine—lacks the methyl substituent in the amino group. Much of the neuronally released norepinephrine reenters the adrenergic neuron: reentry into the cell is accomplished by a specific, active transport system.

Histamine is a naturally occurring substance involved in anaphylaxis and allergic reactions. It is formed by the decarboxylation of histidine and is catabolized by two routes: one involving oxidative deamination with subsequent conjugation with ribose, and the other involving ring methylation with subsequent side-chain oxidation.

Epinephrine is a catecholamine released by the adrenal medulla. It is formed by *N*-methylation of norepinephrine, a reaction catalyzed by the enzyme phenylethanolamine-*N*-methyltransferase. In large part, circulating epinephrine is methylated by catechol-*O*-methyltransferase, and the resultant metanephrine undergoes oxidative deamination by monoamine oxidase to yield 3-methoxy-4-hydroxymandelic acid.

319-321. The answers are: 319-A, 320-C, 321-D. *(Gilman, ed 6. pp 72-73, 615-616, 635-636.)* Epinephrine is made from tyrosine in a series of steps through dopa, dopamine, norepinephrine, and finally epinephrine. The conversion of tyrosine to dopa by tyrosine hydroxylase is the rate-limiting step in this pathway. Epinephrine constitutes about 80 percent of the catecholamines in the adrenal medulla. The enzyme that synthesizes epinephrine from norepinephrine is also found in certain areas of the central nervous system.

Histamine, formed by the decarboxylation of histidine, is stored in mast cells and basophils; some other tissues can synthesize histamine but do not store it. Histamine is released from sensitized mast cells during allergic reactions.

Serotonin (5-hydroxytryptamine) is synthesized from tryptophan in two steps. Tryptophan is hydroxylated by tryptophan hydroxylase, and 5-hydroxytryptophan is decarboxylated to give serotonin. Most serotonin in the body is found in the enterochromaffin cells of the intestinal tract and the pineal gland. Platelets take up and store serotonin but do not synthesize it.

322-327. The answers are: 322-C, 323-E, 324-D, 325-A, 326-D, 327-D. *(Craig, pp 119, 162-163, 172, 176, 198-199, 209.)* Acetylcholine is synthesized from acetyl-CoA and choline. Choline is taken up into the neurons by an active transport system. Hemicholinium blocks this uptake, depleting cellular choline, so that synthesis of acetylcholine no longer occurs.

Botulinus toxin comes from *Clostridium botulinum*, an organism that causes food poisoning. Botulinus toxin prevents the release of acetylcholine from nerve endings, by mechanisms that are not clear. Death occurs from respiratory failure due to the inability of diaphragm muscles to contract.

Tubocurarine is a nondepolarizing agent that binds to the cholinergic receptor at skeletal muscle. It acts as a competitive inhibitor of acetylcholine. Because it is a quaternary ammonium compound, tubocurarine is poorly absorbed from the gastrointestinal tract and is usually given parenterally.

Hexamethonium is also a competitive inhibitor of acetylcholine, but this drug is specific for the nicotinic receptor in the ganglia. Dexamethonium, with 10 carbons instead of 6, is specific for nicotinic receptors at the neuromuscular junction. Hexamethonium causes hypotension by preventing sympathetic constriction of the blood vessels.

Pilocarpine, a plant alkaloid, is a muscarinic agonist. It stimulates sweat glands, salivary glands, and gastric secretions, but it is less effective than acetylcholine in slowing the heart rate. Pilocarpine is used in the treatment of glaucoma to reduce intraocular pressure; by inducing miosis, the drug enhances the outflow of aqueous humor.

Diisopropyl fluorophosphate is an organophosphate inhibitor of acetylcholinesterase that was developed shortly before World War II. Such inhibitors are widely used as insecticides. Diisopropyl fluorophosphate reacts irreversibly with acetylchlolinesterase so that the action of acetylcholine cannot be terminated.

328-331. The answers are: 328-A, 329-C, 330-E, 331-B. *(Gilman, ed 6. pp 92, 129, 793-796, 942-947, 958.)* Methysergide, an ergot alkaloid, is a potent antagonist of 5-hydroxytryptamine in the central nervous system. Unlike most ergot alkaloids, it has no effect on the uterus. Methysergide is used for the prevention of migraine but does not affect an acute attack once it has started.

Methacholine, or acetyl-β-methylcholine, is a choline ester that is hydrolyzed more slowly than acetylcholine by acetylcholinesterase and hydrolyzed to only a slight extent by pseudocholinesterase. The resistance of methacholine to hydrolysis results in a duration of action greater than that of acetylcholine. Methacholine is used to treat acute attacks of narrow-angle glaucoma.

Methyldopa (Aldomet) is one of the major agents used to treat essential hypertension. The antihypertensive effect occurs through the central nervous system. Methyldopa in single oral doses causes a decreased blood pressure characterized by a maximum effect occurring within 4 to 6 hours of ingestion and a hypotensive effect persisting for up to 24 hours after administration. Sedation commonly accompanies treatment.

Methscopolamine is a quaternary amine formed by methylation of the tertiary amine of the naturally occurring scopolamine. It retains the anticholinergic actions of scopolamine but, because of its ionic character, does not penetrate the central nervous system. Because of its anticholinergic inhibition of nasal secretions, methscopolamine is a constituent of cold medications.

Methoxsalen (Oxsoralen) may possibly be effective for chemotherapy of vitiligo, for increasing the tolerance of the skin to sunlight exposure, and for management of psoriasis. Melanocytes must be present for the drug to be effective in vitiligo. Exposure to ultraviolet light causes covalent bonds to form between pyrimidine bases and methoxsalen, which inhibits cell division.

Cardiovascular System

DIRECTIONS: Each question below contains five suggested answers. Choose the **one best** response to each question.

332. Methyldopa (Aldomet) is an antihypertensive agent that acts by

(A) blocking β-adrenergic receptors
(B) preventing conversion of angiotensinogen to angiotensin
(C) altering central sympathetic nervous activity
(D) directly dilating arteriolar smooth muscle
(E) producing catecholamine depletion at postganglionic sympathetic nerve endings

333. Infusion of a small amount of norepinephrine increases all the following cardiovascular parameters EXCEPT

(A) systolic pressure
(B) diastolic pressure
(C) mean pressure
(D) heart rate
(E) peripheral resistance

334. Hypotension resulting from spinal anesthesia can be corrected with

(A) atropine
(B) ephedrine
(C) phentolamine
(D) phenoxybenzamine
(E) reserpine

335. Specificity for the digitalis-induced ventricular tachyarrhythmias associated with acute digitalis intoxication is exhibited by which of the following antiarrhythmic drugs?

(A) Disopyramide (Norpace)
(B) Lidocaine
(C) Procainamide
(D) Propranolol (Inderal)
(E) Quinidine

336. Captopril, an effective agent in treating hypertension, is associated with which of the following side effects?

(A) Postural hypotension
(B) Proteinurea
(C) Hypoglycemia
(D) Hirsutism
(E) Lupus erythematosus-like syndrome

337. Which of the following drugs may enhance rather than suppress ventricular arrhythmias?

(A) Phenytoin (Dilantin)
(B) Isoproterenol (Isuprel)
(C) Lidocaine (Xylocaine)
(D) Procainamide (Pronestyl)
(E) Propranolol (Inderal)

338. The alterations in the electrocardiogram shown below probably resulted from the administration of

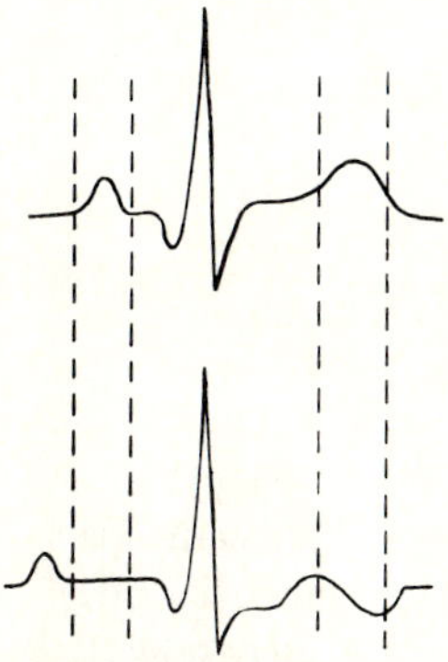

(A) quinidine
(B) lidocaine
(C) digitalis
(D) propranolol
(E) phenytoin

339. A 35-year-old woman who has asthma, coronary insufficiency, and type 2 hyperlipoproteinemia suffers an acute anginal attack. She should be treated with which of the following drugs?

(A) Aminophylline
(B) Nitroglycerin
(C) Papaverine
(D) Propranolol (Inderal)
(E) Sodium nitrite

340. The electrocardiogram of a patient who is receiving digitalis in the therapeutic dose range would be most likely to show

(A) prolongation of the Q-T interval
(B) prolongation of the P-R interval
(C) symmetrical peaking of the T wave
(D) widening of the QRS complex
(E) none of the above

341. A person is likely to be more susceptible to digitoxin toxicity if digitoxin is taken with which of the following drugs?

(A) Neomycin
(B) Hydrochlorothiazide
(C) Phenobarbital
(D) Thioridazine
(E) Estradiol

342. In a hypertensive patient who is taking insulin to treat diabetes, which of the following drugs is contraindicated?

(A) Hydralazine
(B) Prazosin (Minipress)
(C) Guanethidine (Ismelin)
(D) Propranolol (Inderal)
(E) α-Methyldopa (Aldomet)

343. Digoxin is best described by which of the following statements?

(A) Over 90 percent is bound to plasma proteins
(B) It undergoes enterohepatic circulation
(C) It is completely absorbed after oral administration
(D) It is excreted virtually unchanged
(E) It has a high margin of safety

344. A major biochemical effect of cardiac glycosides is

(A) enhancement of cardiac ribosome function in protein synthesis
(B) enhancement of muscarine endplate receptor function in the heart
(C) inhibition of acetylcholinesterase
(D) inhibition of monoamine oxidase
(E) inhibition of Na^+-, K^+-stimulated ATPase

345. If both drugs are administered concurrently, quinidine has which of the following effects on digoxin?

(A) The absorption of digoxin from the GI tract is decreased
(B) The metabolism of digoxin is prevented
(C) The concentration of digoxin in the plasma is increased
(D) The effect of digoxin on the AV node is antagonized
(E) The ability of digoxin to inhibit the Na^+-, K^+-stimulated ATPase is reduced

346. Verapamil exerts its effects through which of the following actions?

(A) Preventing entry of calcium through slow channels
(B) Preventing repolarization of the cell membrane
(C) Increasing sodium entry
(D) Antagonizing the opening of the fast sodium channel
(E) Enhancing potassium efflux

347. The drug of choice for the treatment of a life-threatening hypertensive crisis is

(A) chlorothiazide
(B) diazoxide (Hyperstat)
(C) guanethidine (Ismelin)
(D) methyldopa (Aldomet)
(E) reserpine

348. All the following agents have a central nervous system depressant action EXCEPT

(A) amobarbital (Amytal)
(B) ethyl alcohol
(C) glutethimide
(D) guanethidine (Ismelin)
(E) methaqualone (Quaalude)

349. Blood pressure is directly affected by which of the following peptides?

(A) Renin
(B) Angiotensin I
(C) Angiotensin II
(D) Hageman factor (factor XII)
(E) Kininogen

350. Variations in intestinal absorption, metabolic inactivation, diet, and genetic susceptibility influence the anticoagulant effects of coumarin and indandione anticoagulants. The efficiency of these drugs can best be measured by testing

(A) antihemophilic factor (VIII)
(B) Hageman factor (XII)
(C) Ivy-White bleeding time
(D) partial thromboplastin time
(E) prothrombin time

351. Drugs that are widely used to treat hypertension include all the following EXCEPT

(A) reserpine
(B) hydralazine
(C) chlorothiazide
(D) methyldopa (Aldomet)
(E) glutethimide

352. The antihypertensive effect of guanethidine (Ismelin) is explained by which of the following actions?

(A) Blocking release of intraneuronal catecholamines
(B) Causing direct relaxation of arteriolar smooth muscle
(C) Inhibiting monoamine oxidase
(D) Inhibiting postsynaptic adrenergic receptors
(E) Inhibiting postsynaptic acetylcholine receptors

353. The use of hydralazine in some persons is associated with a sympathetic reflex discharge that may cause tachycardia and arrhythmia. The drug that would be most useful in reducing this reflex stimulation of the heart is

(A) atropine
(B) isoproterenol
(C) procainamide
(D) propranolol (Inderal)
(E) quinidine

354. Hyperlipoproteinemia that is characterized by elevated plasma levels of chylomicrons, normal plasma levels of β lipoproteins, and for which no known drug has proved useful in reducing lipoprotein levels is which of the following types?

(A) Type 1
(B) Type 2
(C) Type 3
(D) Type 4
(E) Type 5

DIRECTIONS: Each question below contains four suggested answers of which **one** or **more** is correct. Choose the answer:

A	if	**1, 2, and 3**	are correct
B	if	**1 and 3**	are correct
C	if	**2 and 4**	are correct
D	if	**4**	is correct
E	if	**1, 2, 3, and 4**	are correct

355. True statements concerning the pharmacologic effects of guanethidine (Ismelin) include which of the following?

(1) It depletes catecholamines from postganglionic adrenergic neurons
(2) Following intravenous administration, it can transiently raise blood pressure by a tyramine-like effect, which can be blocked with cocaine
(3) It has a bretylium-like effect, selectively blocking norepinephrine release in response to activation of postganglionic adrenergic neurons
(4) Like reserpine, it crosses the blood-brain barrier to lower levels of brain amines

356. Clinical effects of therapeutic doses of the benzamide procainamide include

(1) enhancement of intraventricular conduction
(2) ineffectiveness against atrial arrhythmias
(3) occasional production of some symptoms of cinchonism
(4) depression of myocardial contractility

357. β-Adrenergic receptors can be separated into two subclasses—β_1 and β_2 receptors. The β_2 receptors are involved in which of the following adrenergic responses?

(1) Stimulation of myocardial contractility
(2) Relaxation of bronchial smooth muscle
(3) Relaxation of gastrointestinal smooth muscle
(4) Stimulation of renin secretion

358. Isoproterenol modifies the cardiovascular system by interaction mediated via which of the following receptors?

(1) β_2-Adrenergic receptors in the heart
(2) α_1-Adrenergic receptors in arterioles
(3) β_1-Adrenergic receptors in arterioles
(4) β_2-Adrenergic receptors in arterioles

359. Digitalis is given to patients with atrial fibrillation because it

(1) decreases the excitability of the atria
(2) depresses conductivity in the AV node
(3) decreases automaticity of the atria
(4) increases the effective refractory period in the AV node

360. Pure α-adrenergic responses produced by catecholamines include

(1) vasoconstriction
(2) pupillary dilatation
(3) contraction of the splenic capsule
(4) bronchial relaxation

361. Under conditions permitting vagal reflexes, the effects of digitalis on heart tissue include

(1) a shortening of the atrial refractory period
(2) a shortening of the ventricular refractory period
(3) a prolongation of the atrioventricular node refractory period
(4) an increase in rate of contractions

362. Digitalis intoxication may cause which of the following arrhythmias?

(1) Ventricular extrasystole
(2) Partial atrioventricular block
(3) Atrial fibrillation
(4) Ventricular fibrillation

363. In a patient who has early congestive heart failure, which of the following effects could be produced by digitalis therapy?

(1) Increased cardiac output
(2) Diuresis
(3) Decreased heart size
(4) Decreased central venous pressure

364. Relaxation of smooth muscle of both venules and arterioles is produced by which of the following drugs?

(1) Hydralazine
(2) Minoxidil (Loniten)
(3) Diazoxide (Hyperstat)
(4) Sodium nitroprusside

365. People with genetically low levels of *N*-acetyltransferase are more prone to develop a lupus erythematosus-like syndrome with which of the following drugs?

(1) Propranolol (Inderal)
(2) Procainamide
(3) Digitoxin
(4) Hydralazine

366. An anticholinergic, vagolytic effect that can cause an increase in heart rate occurs with which of the following drugs?

(1) Phenytoin (Dilantin)
(2) Procainamide
(3) Lidocaine
(4) Quinidine

367. The automaticity of Purkinje's fibers of the heart can be increased by

(1) epinephrine
(2) quinidine
(3) digitalis
(4) high potassium concentration

SUMMARY OF DIRECTIONS

A	B	C	D	E
1, 2, 3 only	1, 3 only	2, 4 only	4 only	All are correct

368. Pronounced hypotension often occurs after rapid intravenous administration of which of the following drugs?

(1) Lidocaine
(2) Procainamide
(3) Propranolol (Inderal)
(4) Quinidine

369. Fatal arrhythmias are likely to occur in fully digitalized patients who have

(1) hypokalemia
(2) acidosis
(3) hypercalcemia
(4) myocardial infarction

370. Drugs that produce vasodilation by acting directly on vascular smooth muscle include

(1) diazoxide (Hyperstat)
(2) phentolamine
(3) sodium nitroprusside
(4) trimethaphan (Arfonad)

371. Ejaculatory inhibition can result from treatment with

(1) propranolol (Inderal)
(2) chlorothiazide
(3) hydralazine
(4) guanethidine (Ismelin)

372. Cardiotoxic doses of the cardiac glycosides commonly produce

(1) prolonged P-R intervals
(2) enhanced automaticity of Purkinje's fibers
(3) ventricular tachyarrhythmias
(4) enhanced conduction along Purkinje's fibers

373. An increased heart rate is often caused by which of the following drugs?

(1) Propranolol (Inderal)
(2) Reserpine
(3) Methyldopa (Aldomet)
(4) Hydralazine

374. Hyperlipidemia can be treated by which of the following agents?

(1) Clofibrate (Atromid-S)
(2) Cholestyramine (Questran)
(3) Nicotinic acid
(4) Propylthiouracil

375. Megaloblastic anemia is associated with which of the following findings?

(1) A deficiency of intrinsic factor
(2) An arrest of maturation in the erythroid cells in the bone marrow
(3) Hypersegmentation of the nuclei of polymorphonuclear leukocytes
(4) Microcytic anemia

376. Megaloblastic anemia may be responsive to administration of

(1) cyanocobalamin
(2) intrinsic factor concentrate
(3) folic acid
(4) ferrous sulfate

377. Endogenous heparin is characterized by which of the following statements?

(1) It is found largely in mast cells
(2) It is a sulfonated mucopolysaccharide
(3) It is inhibited by protamine sulfate
(4) It is able to release a lipemia-clearing factor

378. Clofibrate (Atromid-S) is associated with which of the following side effects?

(1) Myopathy
(2) Potentiation of coumarin anticoagulants
(3) Gallbladder disease
(4) Cholestatic jaundice

379. In the treatment of hypertension, hydralazine is rarely given alone because it

(1) increases cardiac output through reflex sympathetic stimulation
(2) causes severe postural hypotension
(3) elevates plasma renin levels
(4) compromises the metabolism of other drugs

380. β-Adrenergic blocking agents are useful for treating which of the following conditions?

(1) Hypertension
(2) Angina pectoris
(3) Supraventricular tachycardia
(4) Congestive heart failure

DIRECTIONS: The groups of questions below consist of lettered choices followed by several numbered items. For each numbered item select the **one** lettered choice with which it is **most** closely associated. Each lettered choice may be used once, more than once, or not at all.

Questions 381-384

For each drug that follows, select the mechanism of action that is most appropriate.

(A) Binds bile acids in the intestine
(B) Decreases cholesterol synthesis and lipoprotein release from the liver
(C) Inhibits free fatty acid release from adipose tissue
(D) Promotes hepatic conversion of cholesterol to bile acids
(E) Promotes renal excretion of cholesterol and triglycerides

381. Cholestyramine (Questran)
382. Clofibrate (Atromid-S)
383. Dextrothyroxine (Choloxin)
384. Nicotinic acid

Questions 385-389

Match each route of administration and treatment indication with the correct drug.

(A) Isoproterenol
(B) Terbutaline
(C) Phenylephrine
(D) Dextroamphetamine sulfate (Dexedrine)
(E) Prazosin (Minipress)

385. Administered intravenously to terminate paroxysmal atrial tachycardia
386. Administered parenterally to produce myocardial stimulation
387. Administered orally in the treatment of narcolepsy
388. Administered topically as a nasal decongestant
389. Administered orally to produce bronchodilation

Questions 390-394

For each description that follows, choose the antiarrhythmic drug with which is it most likely to be associated.

(A) Lidocaine
(B) Propranolol (Inderal)
(C) Quinidine
(D) Procainamide
(E) Phenytoin (Dilantin)

B 390. Blocks the effects of catecholamines upon the heart

D 391. Can cause a syndrome resembling lupus erythematosus

A 392. Is usually given intravenously but can also be given intramuscularly

C 393. A naturally occurring substance

A 394. Is not recommended for the treatment of supraventricular arrhythmias

Questions 395-399

Match the following.

(A) Inhibits thrombin and early coagulation steps
(B) Inhibits synthesis of prothrombin
(C) Inhibits platelet aggregation
(D) Activates plasminogen
(E) Binds the calcium ion cofactor in some coagulation steps

B 395. Coumarin

C 396. Dipyridamole

E 397. Ethylenediaminetetraacetic acid (EDTA)

A 398. Heparin

D 399. Streptokinase

Questions 400-404

Match the following.

(A) Angiotensin I
(B) Angiotensin II
(C) Clonidine
(D) Saralasin
(E) Captopril

B 400. Formed by sequential enzymatic cleavage by renin and then peptidyl dipeptidase (kinase II)

D 401. An octapeptide that lowers blood pressure in renin-dependent hypertensive patients

E 402. Lowers blood pressure in hypertensive patients by inhibiting peptidyl dipeptidase

A 403. Cleaves to a pressor octapeptide on single passage through the lungs

B 404. An octapeptide that is a potent vasoconstrictor

Cardiovascular System

Answers

332. The answer is C. *(Craig, pp 364-365.)* Methyldopa (Aldomet) is frequently used to treat hypertension. It exerts an antihypertensive effect by acting through the central nervous system. Methyldopa is metabolized to α-methylnorepinephrine after it is taken up by nerve endings. The action of this metabolite on α-adrenergic receptors in the brain is thought to account for methyldopa's effect.

333. The answer is D. *(Goth, ed 10. p 180.)* On infusion of a small amount of norepinephrine, the heart rate may become slightly decreased. Systolic, diastolic, and mean pressures, as well as peripheral resistance, will increase. The elevated blood pressure causes a reflex increase in vagal tone and a slowing of the heart rate. This slowing may be blocked with atropine.

334. The answer is B. *(Gilman, ed 6. pp 169, 315.)* The hypotension that occurs during spinal anesthesia is a result of loss of sympathetic tone. To correct this condition, ephedrine and mephentermine are the drugs of choice because they produce vasoconstriction without causing such severe increases in peripheral vascular resistance that the heart may fail. These drugs should be used only if postural changes to correct the hypotension are ineffective. The hypotension associated with general anesthesias, such as cyclopropane and halothane, is not treated with sympathomimetics, however, because these anesthetic agents sensitize the heart to the arrhythmogenic effects of the sympathomimetics.

335. The answer is B. *(Gilman, ed 6. pp 769, 779-780.)* Lidocaine neither depresses the excitability, nor prolongs the effective refractory period, of the atrium, ventricle, or specialized conduction system. Depressed conduction through the AV node occurs during digitalis toxicity. Thus, lidocaine provides significant benefits in comparison with the antiarrhythmic agents quinidine, procainamide, disopyramide (Norpace), and propranolol (Inderal).

336. The answer is B. *(Craig, pp 376-377.)* Captopril inhibits angiotensin-converting enzyme, which converts angiotensin I to the vasoconstrictor angiotensin II. It also inhibits breakdown of the vasodilator bradykinin. Captopril lacks many side effects of other hypertensive agents; however, about 1 percent of patients taking this drug develop proteinuria, and some of these patients develop a nephrotic syndrome.

337. The answer is B. *(Craig, pp 127, 221-228.)* Isoproterenol (Isuprel) is a sympathomimetic agent that stimulates chiefly β receptors and that can induce ventricular tachycardia and other arrhythmias. All the other drugs listed in the question are, in therapeutic doses, antiarrhythmic agents. However, in large doses, phenytoin (Dilantin) may elicit various arrhythmias, and propranolol (Inderal) may produce bradyarrhythmia.

338. The answer is C. *(Gilman, ed 6. pp 742, 768.)* The Q-T interval of an electrocardiogram may be shortened by administration of lidocaine, digitalis, and phenytoin. Of these, digitalis is the most likely to increase the P-R interval. The electrocardiographic manifestations of digitalis initially include diminished T-wave amplitude and biphasia, with ST depression. P-R interval prolongation occurs later than these changes, and a P-R interval prolongation of about 0.20 seconds (borderline first-degree AV block) may be an indication of digitalis intoxication. A decreased Q-T interval is another effect of digitalis administration and is a consequence of a reduced duration of ventricular systole. The Q-T interval is characteristically prolonged by quinidine and propranolol.

339. The answer is B. *(Craig, pp 286-289, 470.)* Nitroglycerin is the drug of choice for acute anginal attack. The antianginal effect of nitroglycerin derives from its ability to dilate blood vessels in the peripheral circulation, thereby decreasing the volume of blood returning to the heart. Papaverine, a coronary vasodilator, is not as effective as nitroglycerin in relief of angina. Propranolol may induce bronchoconstriction and precipitate an asthmatic attack through β blockade. Aminophylline can reduce the frequency and intensity of an asthmatic attack, but, because aminophylline stimulates the heart, it is of no help in angina. Although the relaxation of smooth muscle is the fundamental pharmacologic action of nitrites, the administration of sodium nitrite is now considered obsolete except for treatment of cyanide poisoning.

340. The answer is B. *(Gilman, ed 6. pp 735, 741-742.)* The usual electrocardiographic pattern of a patient receiving therapeutic doses of digitalis includes an increase in the P-R interval, depression and sagging of the ST segment, and occasional biphasia or inversion of the T wave. Symmetrically peaked T waves are associated with hyperkalemia or ischemia in most cases. Q-T interval shortening, rather than prolongation, is characteristic of digitalis treatment.

341. The answer is B. *(Gilman, ed 6. pp 753, 878.)* Low body stores of potassium increase susceptibility to digitalis toxicity. The thiazide diuretics, such as hydrochlorothiazide, promote excretion of potassium. Diuretics are often given with digitoxin to treat congestive heart failure; this combination frequently causes digitalis toxicity.

342. The answer is D. *(Gilman, ed 6. pp 193-194.)* Propranolol blocks the action of catecholamines at β-adrenergic receptors. It enhances the hypoglycemic effects of insulin because it blocks stimulation of glycogenolysis through β receptors. In addition, the drug masks the symptoms of hypoglycemia, such as sweating and tachycardia. Therefore, propranolol should be used with caution in diabetic patients.

343. The answer is D. *(Gilman, ed 6. pp 746-751.)* Digoxin is a cardiac glycoside commonly used for congestive heart failure. The absorption of preparations taken orally may vary from 40 to 90 percent, depending on the type used. This is an important consideration because of the small margin of safety for this drug—only 2- to 3-fold. About 25 percent of digoxin in the serum is bound to plasma proteins. The drug is excreted almost entirely unchanged by the kidney.

344. The answer is E. *(Craig, p 272.)* A major biochemical effect of cardiac glycosides is the inhibition of Na^+-, K^+-stimulated ATPase, which is thought to be a component of the sodium-potassium pump. This inhibition produces an increase in intracellular sodium and the loss of intracellular potassium. The cardiac disturbances that occur in digitalis intoxication may be, in part, related to these electrolyte changes.

345. The answer is C. *(Craig, pp 279-280. Gilman, ed 6. pp 755-756.)* Quinidine is sometimes given in addition to digoxin to treat supraventricular arrhythmias. Quinidine displaces digoxin from skeletal muscle binding sites and may also inhibit excretion of digoxin by the kidneys. As a result, digoxin concentrations in the plasma may increase to toxic levels.

346. The answer is A. *(Craig, pp 223, 265-266.)* Verapamil is used to treat angina and supraventricular tachyarrhythmias. It acts by suppressing calcium entry through the slow calcium channel of the heart but does not affect the rapid entry of sodium. The inward current in the AV node is primarily through the slow calcium channel, and, therefore, verapamil slows conduction through the AV node.

347. The answer is B. *(Craig, pp 348-349.)* Diazoxide, given intravenously, is a rapidly acting vasodilator. It is the preferred drug for a hypertensive crisis. The onset of action of the other drugs listed in the question is considerably longer than for diazoxide; they are more useful for the chronic control of hypertension or the subacute stabilization of patients for whom chemotherapy was initiated with diazoxide.

348. The answer is D. *(Gilman, ed 6. pp 199, 351, 364, 367, 376.)* Owing to its inability readily to pass the blood-brain barrier, the antihypertensive agent guanethidine (Ismelin) has negligible effect on the central nervous system. Amobarbital, ethyl alcohol, glutethimide, and methaqualone are used for their hypnotic or sedative actions and readily cross the blood-brain barrier. Investigators generally consider lipid solubility to be the factor that directly determines the capacity of drugs to enter the central nervous system. Guanethidine—a strong base—lacks lipid solubility and diminishes responses to activated adrenergic nerves.

349. The answer is C. *(Gilman, ed 6. pp 660-661.)* Renin hydrolyzes plasma angiotensin precursor to angiotensin I, the inactive precursor of angiotensin II, a potent, direct-acting vasoconstrictor. Hageman factor is the precursor of prekallikrein activator and does not have a direct vasoactive effect. Kallikrein is the enzyme that converts kininogen to bradykinin, a vasodilator. The pharmacologic effects of angiotensin II include elevation of blood pressure, release of aldosterone leading to retention of sodium, and the release of catecholamines.

350. The answer is E. *(Gilman, ed 6. pp 1354, 1358. Goth, ed 10. pp 482-483.)* The best measure of the efficiency of coumarin as an anticoagulant is prothrombin time, which is greatly prolonged following the administration of coumarin and indandione derivatives due to their suppressing the formation of prothrombin and factors II, VII, IX, and X. The synthesis of factors VIII and XII is not inhibited by these agents. When therapy with these anticoagulants is discontinued, blood prothrombin time returns to normal in one to eight days.

351. The answer is E. *(Craig, pp 338-340, 345-347, 361, 364-365.)* Glutethimide is a sedative-hypnotic drug that is not customarily employed, even in adjunctive therapy of hypertension. Chlorothiazide reduces hypertension through its diuretic action. Hydralazine reduces peripheral arteriolar resistance and elicits reflex tachycardia. Methyldopa (Aldomet) exerts its chief antihypertensive action on the central nervous system (CNS), and reserpine acts both on the CNS and at the site of adrenergic neurons.

352. The answer is A. *(Gilman, ed 6. pp 198-199.)* Guanethidine (Ismelin) prevents release of norepinephrine from nerve endings when the nerves are stimulated. The drug must be taken up by the nerves to exert its effects. Although guanethidine causes depletion of norepinephrine, this depletion is not the primary effect and is incidental to the antihypertensive action of guanethidine.

353. The answer is D. *(Craig, pp 345-347.)* Hydralazine causes peripheral vasodilatation that in some patients is associated with a sympathetic reflex discharge causing disturbances in cardiac rate and rhythm. Propranolol (Inderal) is considered the drug of choice to reduce this reflex stimulation of the heart. Its β-blocking effect slows the heart rate and prevents ectopic rhythms. Atropine would produce tachycardia by its vagolytic effect. Isoproterenol, the most active of the sympathomimetic amines, acts strongly on all β receptors and would directly affect the heart chronotropically and inotropically, often in association with atrial and ventricular tachycardia and ectopic rhythms. Quinidine and procainamide are antiarrhythmic agents of no use in treating reflex (sympathetic) tachycardia.

354. The answer is A. *(Craig, pp 301-303. Gilman, ed 6. pp 837-838.)* In type 1 hyperlipoproteinemia, drugs that reduce levels of lipoproteins are not useful, but reduction of dietary sources of fat may help. Maintenance of ideal body weight is recommended in all types of hyperlipidemia. Clofibrate (Atromid-S) effectively reduces the levels of very-low density lipoproteins characteristic of types 3, 4, and 5 hyperlipoproteinemias; and administration of cholestyramine resin, in conjunction with a low-cholesterol diet, is regarded as effective therapy for type 2a, or primary hyperbetalipoproteinemia, except in the homozygous familial form.

355. The answer is A (1, 2, 3). *(Craig, pp 359-360. Gilman, ed 6. pp 198-199.)* Unlike reserpine, guanethidine (Ismelin) cannot cross the blood-brain barrier in sufficient amounts to affect levels of brain amines. Its basic ionic structure is the pharmacologic basis for this failure to reach the central nervous system. Like reserpine, guanethidine causes the depletion of catecholamines; but, like tyramine, this widely used hypertensive drug can cause the release of catecholamines. Guanethidine's ability to block selectively the release of norepinephrine in response to the activation of postganglionic neurons is similar to that of bretylium.

356. The answer is C (2, 4). *(Craig, pp 230, 232, 234-238.)* Procainamide retards rather than enhances intraventricular conduction, an effect that is expressed as a widening of the QRS complex of the electrocardiogram. Although not always effective in the treatment of atrial arrhythmias, procainamide is useful in some patients. Long-term administration of procainamide commonly causes a syndrome similar to systemic lupus erythematosus. The degree of hypotension that results from intravenous infusion of procainamide is greater following rapid, compared to slow, administration. The hypotensive effect, less marked after intramuscular injection and absent after oral administration, is considered to be the result of both vasodilation and depression of myocardial contractility. Quinidine, in large doses, can cause an adverse effect called cinchonism, a cluster of symptoms that includes tinnitus, headache, nausea, and disturbances in hearing and vision.

357. The answer is C (2, 4). *(Gilman, ed 6. pp 60-61.)* Relaxation of bronchial and vascular smooth muscle by β-adrenergic stimulants involves β_2 receptors. Renin secretion is also stimulated by β_2 receptors. Stimulation of myocardial contractility involves β_1 receptors.

358. The answer is D (4). *(Gilman, ed 6. pp 153-154.)* Isoproterenol is the most active of the selective β-sympathomimetic agents. It has virtually no α activity, yet it manifests potent cardiac inotropic and chronotropic (β_1) as well as vasodilator and bronchodilator (β_2) activity.

359. The answer is C (2, 4). *(Craig, pp 273-277. Gilman, ed 6. pp 739-740, 750.)* Digitalis is used in atrial fibrillation to slow the ventricular rate; the atrial fibrillation itself is not usually controlled. Digitalis acts to slow the speed of conduction and to increase the effective refractory period in the AV node, which prevents transmission of all the impulses from the atria to the ventricles. The drug exerts these effects on the AV node by direct action on the heart and by indirectly increasing vagal activity.

360. The answer is A (1, 2, 3). *(Gilman, ed 6. pp 60-61, 165.)* α-Adrenergic responses include vasoconstriction, pupillary dilatation, and contraction of the nictitating membrane and splenic capsule. β-Adrenergic responses include bronchial relaxation, vasodilatation (in skeletal muscle), gastrointestinal hypomotility, and cardiac chronotropic as well as inotropic stimulation. Catecholamines with pure α-adrenergic effects include phenylephrine and methoxamine (Vasoxyl).

361. The answer is A (1, 2, 3). *(Craig, pp 274-275. Gilman, ed 6. pp 737-745.)* Digitalis shortens the atrial and ventricular refractory periods and prolongs the functional refractory period of the AV node. This prolongation of the functional refractory period of the AV node is employed in the control of supraventricular tachycardias. Heart rate is decreased through vagal and direct effects of digitalis, effects that are more pronounced in the failing than normal heart. In the absence of vagal effects, the abbreviation of atrial refractory period and the prolongation of AV nodal functional refractory period are both much less pronounced.

362. The answer is E (all). *(Gilman, ed 6. pp 751-753.)* Although ventricular extrasystole is a common arrhythmia associated with digitalis therapy, all the arrhythmias listed in the question may occur in digitalis intoxication. Ventricular fibrillation is the most common cause of death in patients who become toxic to digitalis. Other consequences of digitalis intoxication include: blurred, "frosted," or "white" vision; neuralgia (particularly trigeminal); malaise, anorexia, and nausea with vomiting; and (only rarely) rashes, eosinophilia, and gynecomastia.

363. The answer is E (all). *(Gilman, ed 6. pp 743-746.)* Digitalis therapy in early congestive heart failure directly enhances myocardial contractility and increases cardiac output. These effects on the myocardium and cardiac output decrease heart size and end-diastolic volume and lower central venous pressure. Diuresis is accomplished indirectly through enhanced renal perfusion and glomerular filtration.

364. The answer is D (4). *(Craig, pp 345-350.)* Hydralazine, minoxidil, diazoxide, and sodium nitroprusside are all directly acting vasodilators used to treat hypertension. Because hydralazine, minoxidil, and diazoxide relax arteriolar smooth muscle more than smooth muscle in venules, the effect on venous capacitance is negligible. Sodium nitroprusside, which affects both arterioles and venules, does not increase cardiac output, a feature that enhances the utility of sodium nitroprusside in the management of hypertensive crisis associated with myocardial infarction.

365. The answer is C (2, 4). *(Gilman, ed 6. pp 775, 801.)* Individuals with low hepatic *N*-acetyltransferase activity are known as slow acetylators. A major pathway of metabolism of both procainamide, used to treat arrhythmias, and hydralazine, used to prevent hypertension, is *N*-acetylation. Slow acetylators receiving these drugs are more susceptible than normal persons to side effects, since slow acetylators will have higher than normal blood levels of these drugs. *N*-Acetylprocainamide, the metabolite of procainamide, is also active, and is being tested as an antiarryhthmic agent.

366. The answer is C (2, 4). *(Craig, pp 229-231.)* Therapy with quinidine and procainamide is associated with vagolytic effects that do not occur during therapy with phenytoin (Dilantin) and lidocaine. Disorders of impulse formation constitute a mechanism that is generally considered to cause most tachyarrhythmias and that can be abolished by administration of quinidine, which–like procainamide–decreases the rate of diastolic depolarization and increases the threshold of myocardial excitability. However, the direct, or antiarrhythmic, effect of quinidine is opposed by its vagolytic effect, which may lead to tachycardia.

367. The answer is B (1, 3). *(Gilman, ed 6. pp 147, 734, 768.)* Automaticity of Purkinje's fibers is increased by epinephrine, digitalis, isoproterenol, and low potassium concentration. It is decreased by quinidine or high potassium concentration. The modification of automaticity is important: in complete heart block, a condition of rhythm failure with bradycardia, isoproterenol or epinephrine might be used to enhance lower conductive system automaticity. However, in the situation of supraventricular and ventricular ectopy, all agents able to facilitate automaticity should be avoided.

368. The answer is C (2, 4). *(Craig, p 232.)* Procainamide and quinidine are potent vasodilators and thus tend to lower arterial pressure. High concentrations of these drugs also depress myocardial contractility; in some cases, the decrease in cardiac output contributes to the hypotension, especially in the presence of myocardial damage. The effects of lidocaine and propranolol (Inderal) on arterial pressure are much less obvious.

369. The answer is E (all). *(Gilman, ed 6. pp 753-754.)* Fatal cardiac arrhythmias are likely to occur in fully digitalized patients who have myocardial infarction, hypoxia, acid-base imbalances, hypercalcemia, hypomagnesemia, or hypokalemia, the last condition generally regarded as being the most frequent cause of digitalis intoxication. The actions of digitalis upon the Na^+-, K^+-ATPase pump provide a molecular basis for the toxicity enhancement due to low potassium and high calcium concentrations. Acidosis and ischemia are deleterious to the heart in a more general way, but they also may deplete intracellular potassium and so enhance toxicity.

370. The answer is B (1, 3). *(Craig, pp 199-200, 348-350.)* Both diazoxide (Hyperstat), which is chemically related to but pharmacologically distinct from the thiazide diuretics, and sodium nitroprusside (or sodium nitroferricyanide) are potent, directly acting vasodilators that are given intravenously in hypertensive emergencies. In pharmacodynamic studies of hypertensive patients, diazoxide has been shown to dilate arterioles to a far greater degree than large veins, increase cardiac output without functional impairment of the sympathetic nervous system, and act principally on resistance rather than capacitance vessels. However, sodium nitroprusside acts on both resistance and capacitance vessels and, compared to diazoxide, is more likely to induce postural hypotension. Trimethaphan (Arfonad) is also used parenterally for the same purpose; but it produces vasodilation secondary to a decrease in sympathetic tone, which results from the blockade of transmission through sympathetic ganglia. Phentolamine causes vasodilation by blocking the α receptors, preventing vasoconstriction caused by the sympathetic nervous system.

371. The answer is D (4). *(Craig, pp 359-360.)* Hypertensive patients who are receiving therapeutic doses of guanethidine (Ismelin), which selectively depresses the function of postganglionic adrenergic nerves, commonly experience an inhibition of ejaculation—basically a spinal reflex that involves adrenergic fibers. Impotence can be a psychologic consequence of failure to ejaculate.

372. The answer is A (1, 2, 3). *(Gilman, ed 6. pp 734-742.)* The electrocardiographic manifestations in digitalis intoxication include atrioventricular block and ventricular extrasystoles, tachycardia, and fibrillation. Enhanced automaticity of Purkinje's fibers may be a causative factor in the arrhythmias induced by these drugs. **Conduction** along Purkinje's fibers, however, is depressed, not enhanced.

373. The answer is D (4). *(Gilman, ed 6. pp 191, 203, 795, 799-800.)* Hydralazine, a peripheral vasodilator, lowers arterial pressure and causes an increase in heart rate. (The increase in heart rate is, in part, a reflex caused by low blood pressure.) Propranolol (Inderal) decreases the heart rate by blocking the β-adrenergic cardiac receptors. Reserpine, which depletes adrenergic neurons of norepinephrine, and methyldopa (Aldomet), which lowers sympathetic tone by a mechanism that is unclear, both decrease the heart rate in patients who are being treated for hypertension.

374. The answer is A (1, 2, 3). *(Gilman, ed 6. pp 839-845.)* Clofibrate (Atromid-S), cholestyramine (Questran), and nicotinic acid all have been employed in the treatment of hyperlipidemia. Propylthiouracil decreases the secretion of thyroid hormone, which elevates cholesterol levels in the blood. Nicotinic acid may be used in hyperlipoproteinemia types II, III, IV, and V. Clofibrate is useful in patients with type III; cholestyramine should be used to treat type II.

375. The answer is A (1, 2, 3). *(Gilman, ed 6. p 1336. Isselbacher, ed 9. p 1523.)* Megaloblastic anemia can result from lack of the intrinsic factor that is secreted by normal gastric mucosa and binds vitamin B_{12} (extrinsic factor) to facilitate the absorption of the vitamin by the small intestine. The lack of B_{12} causes a buildup of cells in the DNA doubling stage—an apparent maturation arrest of erythroid elements in the bone marrow—and the appearance in the peripheral blood of white blood cells with hypersegmented nuclei. A microcytic anemia is associated with iron deficiency. In the therapy of megaloblastic anemia, the determination of the existence of a B_{12} deficiency is important because folic acid therapy can correct most of the hematologic abnormalities—although the neurologic damage in B_{12} deficiency will progress.

376. The answer is A (1, 2, 3). *(Gilman, ed 6. pp 1334-1338, 1342-1343.)* Vitamin B_{12} deficiency has several causes. Pernicious anemia, associated with gastric mucosal atrophy and histamine-refractory achlorhydria, eliminates the production of intrinsic factor that would combine with cyanocobalamin (B_{12}) in the gut. Parenteral administration of B_{12} is recommended for patients who have pernicious anemia. Oral B_{12} and intrinsic factor concentrate should be used only in patients who have a proved intrinsic factor deficit and refuse intramuscular administration of B_{12}. Other causes of vitamin B_{12} deficiency, in the face of normal intrinsic factor secretion, include malabsorption syndromes and parasitic competition. Alcohol-associated megaloblastic anemia is usually caused by a deficiency of folic acid.

377. The answer is E (all). *(Gilman, ed 6. pp 1349-1350.)* Heparin, a naturally occurring anticoagulant, is localized largely in mast cells. A mucopolysaccharide, it is composed of sulfated glucosamine and glucuronic acid. Its primary action is as an antithrombin factor, for which it requires a plasma cofactor. Organic bases (protamine) are believed to inhibit heparin by neutralizing its electronegative charge. Heparin is thought to release, and become a part of, a lipemia-clearing factor that catalyzes the hydrolsis of triglycerides.

378. The answer is A (1, 2, 3). *(Craig, p 302. Gilman, ed 6. pp 840-841.)* Clofibrate (Atromid-S) has been noted to cause severe muscle cramps and weakness and to potentiate coumarin anticoagulants, possibly by competing for binding sites in serum albumin. The cause of the myopathy is unknown. Clofibrate stimulates secretion of cholesterol into the bile and increases formation of gallstones, which accounts for the increased incidence of gallbladder disease in persons taking this drug.

379. The answer is B (1, 3). *(Craig, pp 343-347.)* Vasodilation caused by hydralazine results in reflex sympathetic cardiac output, increased plasma renin activity, and decreased sodium excretion. These three factors, all of which result in increased blood pressure, limit the use of vasodilators alone to treat hypertension. To avoid these effects, hydralazine is usually given in combination with propranolol and a diuretic.

380. The answer is A (1, 2, 3). *(Craig, pp 250-256, 290-293, 356-358.)* β-Adrenergic blocking agents such as propranolol (Inderal) have been shown to be useful in treating hypertension, angina pectoris, and supraventricular arrhythmias. β Blockers may cause bronchoconstriction by inhibition of β_2 receptors in the lungs; thus, these drugs are contraindicated in patients suffering from asthma. More selective blockers such as metroprolol (Lopressor), which has a higher affinity for β_1 receptors, are sometimes used, but at high concentrations these drugs can also block β_2 receptors. In congestive heart failure, the heart is under sympathetic control and blocking this stimulation can exacerbate the condition.

381-384. The answers are: 381-A, 382-B, 383-D, 384-C. *(Gilman, ed 6. pp 839-845.)* Cholestyramine (Questran), an anion-exchange resin used to treat hyperbetalipoproteinemia, binds bile acids in the intestine, increasing fecal excretion of the acids.

Clofibrate (Atromid-S) is a cholesterol-synthesis inhibitor that also increases the excretion of neutral sterols. Clofibrate is used to treat several hyperlipidemias, chiefly types 3, 4, and 5, which are characterized by elevated levels of very-low density lipoproteins (VLDL). Sufficient evidence exists to identify clofibrate as an effective agent that can decrease the plasma level of triglycerides by decreasing the concentration of VLDL within two to five days after the first dose.

Thyroid hormones such as dextrothyroxine (Choloxin) have major effects on lipid metabolism: they enhance cholesterol synthesis, increase the conversion of cholesterol to bile acids, and increase the excretion of sterol in the feces.

Nicotinic acid acts by mechanisms that, although largely unknown, include decreased lipolysis and decreased synthesis of low density lipoprotein. Nicotinic acid is effective in all hyperlipidemias except type 1.

385-389. The answers are: 385-C, 386-A, 387-D, 388-C, 389-B. *(Gilman, ed 6. pp 154, 160-161, 165, 167-168, 807.)* Isoproterenol, a catecholamine that acts on β-adrenergic receptors, is given parenterally because absorption after sublingual or oral administrations is unreliable. A synthetic sympathomimetic structurally similar to epinephrine, isoproterenol produces myocardial stimulation and is used for treatment of atrioventricular heart block, cardiogenic shock associated with myocardial infarction, cardiac arrest, and septicemic shock.

Terbutaline is a synthetic sympathomimetic amine that acts on the β_2-adrenergic receptors of bronchial smooth muscle, resulting in a decrease in airway and pulmonary resistance. Oral doses are effective for management of bronchial asthma and for the reversible bronchospasm that may occur in bronchitis and emphysema.

Phenylephrine powerfully stimulates α-adrenergic receptors: its topical administration results in the constriction of the blood vessels of the nasal mucosa, "shrinks" the tissue, and relieves the nasal congestion; its intravenous administration to patients who have paroxysmal atrial tachycardia results in increased arterial pressure (which, in turn, leads to a reflex vagal discharge that terminates the tachycardia).

Dextroamphetamine sulfate (Dexedrine), the racemic form of amphetamine that is about four times more potent than the *l* isomer, is a sympathomimetic noncatecholamine having marked effects upon the central nervous system and generally is preferred for therapy of narcolepsy. It stimulates the medullary respiratory center, decreases the intensity of central nervous sytem depression caused by other drugs, and stimulates the cerebrospinal axis. Oral administration of dextroamphetamine promotes wakefulness and diminishes the amplitude and duration of the delta wave pattern that typically is present during narcolepsy.

Prazosin (Minipress) is an α-adrenergic blocking agent selective for postsynaptic receptors. It is orally administered to treat hypertension; however, the full range of its therapeutic uses, mechanisms of action, and toxicity have not been determined.

390-394. The answers are: 390-B, 391-D, 392-A, 393-C, 394-A. *(Craig, pp 233, 237, 243, 245, 250.)* Propranolol (Inderal) is a β_1- and β_2-adrenergic receptor antagonist used in the treatment of arrhythmias, especially those associated with increased levels of catecholamines. By blocking the action of catecholamines, propranolol induces negative chronotropism and inotropism and reduces the myocardial requirement for oxygen. Other therapeutic indications for propranolol include angina pectoris and, in combination with other drugs, hypertension (except hypertensive crises).

Quinidine, which is isolated from the bark of some species of the South American *Cinchona* tree, is a widely used antiarrhythmic agent that, like procainamide, is useful in the treatment of both supraventricular and ventricular arrhythmias. It should not be given intravenously because the possibility of toxic effects is increased by this route of administration. Toxic effects include myocardial depression and AV block.

Procainamide, an antiarrhythmic agent used to treat both supraventricular and ventricular arrhythmias, has a relatively short biologic half-life that makes frequent, large, oral doses necessary. It has a spectrum of action similar to quinidine, but unlike quinidine, may be given intraventricularly. Its long-term use in certain patients has been cited as a factor causing a syndrome resembling lupus erythematosus.

Lidocaine, widely used as a local anesthetic, also is used for the treatment of ventricular arrhythmias, especially those associated with myocardial infarction. It is also the best drug to use in arrhythmias caused by digitalis intoxication. It has only small effects on the atria and, therefore, is not useful in supraventricular arrhythmias. Because of its very brief biologic half-life, lidocaine is not administered orally for the treatment of arrhythmias; its clinical use is limited to intramuscular and intravenous administration.

395-399. The answers are: 395-B, 396-C, 397-E, 398-A, 399-D. *(Gilman, ed 6. pp 1349-1355, 1361-1362, 1620.)* Heparin's action as an antithrombin factor requires the presence of an α_2 globulin called antithrombin III. Antithrombin III is a protease inhibitor that inhibits the activity of several of the clotting factors by forming irreversible complexes. Heparin facilitates the formation of these complexes and is antagonized by protamine sulfate.

Coumarin, an oral anticoagulant, antagonizes vitamin K and causes a decrease in production of prothrombin and coagulation factors VII, IX, and X. Oral anticoagulants prevent formation of these factors by blocking formation of the reduced form of vitamin K.

Dipyridamole is classified as a coronary vasodilator. Its effectiveness in inhibiting platelet aggregation and adhesion has been proven in vitro but has still to be demonstrated in vivo.

Both urokinase and streptokinase activate plasminogen to plasmin, which is a protease. Plasmin dissolves thrombin by breaking down fibrin.

Ethylenediaminetetraacetic acid (EDTA) inactivates calcium in vitro by forming a complex with the calcium, thus preventing clotting. This approach is impossible in vivo because calcium levels that are low enough to prevent coagulation also are low enough to be lethal.

400-404. The answers are: 400-B, 401-D, 402-E, 403-A, 404-B. *(Gilman, ed 6. pp 647-659, 797-798, 811-813.)* The enzyme, renin, acts upon angiotensinogen (an α globulin) to yield the decapeptide, angiotensin I, which has limited pharmacological activity. Angiotensin I is metabolized extensively in a single passage through the lungs by the carboxypeptidase, peptidyl dipeptidase (also called kinase II or angiotensin-converting enzyme) to the octapeptide, angiotensin II.

Angiotensin II has a potent direct action on the vascular smooth muscle and also indirectly stimulates contraction by means of the sympathetic nervous system. The vasoconstriction in response to angiotensin II involves precapillary arterioles and postcapillary venules and results in an increased total peripheral resistance.

The octapeptide, saralasin, is an analog of angiotensin II and has an alanine in place of the phenylalanine in the 8 position. It is a potent antagonist of angiotensin II and, thus, can reduce elevated blood pressure in individuals with significant amounts of circulating angiotensin II (i.e., renin-dependent hypertension). Being a polypeptide, saralasin must be administered intravenously, which limits its therapeutic use.

Captopril and clonidine, in contrast, are orally effective antihypertensive agents. Captopril (D-3-mercapto-methylpropanoyl-L-proline) is a rationally designed, competitive inhibitor of peptidyl dipeptidase. Unlike saralasin, it blocks the formation but not the response of angiotensin II. Captopril is useful in reducing the blood pressure of both renin-dependent and normal-renin essential hypertension. The hypotensive action of clonidine is believed to be due primarily to stimulation of the α-adrenergic receptors in the central nervous system (CNS). A reduction in the discharge rate of preganglionic adrenergic nerves occurs in addition to bradycardia. The CNS actions of clonidine also lead to a reduction in the level of renin activity in the plasma.

Renal System

DIRECTIONS: Each question below contains five suggested answers. Choose the **one best** response to each question.

405. A form of Fanconi's syndrome may be caused by outdated preparations of which of the following antibiotics?

(A) Gentamicin
(B) Penicillin V
(C) Tetracycline
(D) Erythromycin
(E) Chloramphenicol

406. The structure shown below is a member of which of the following drug groups?

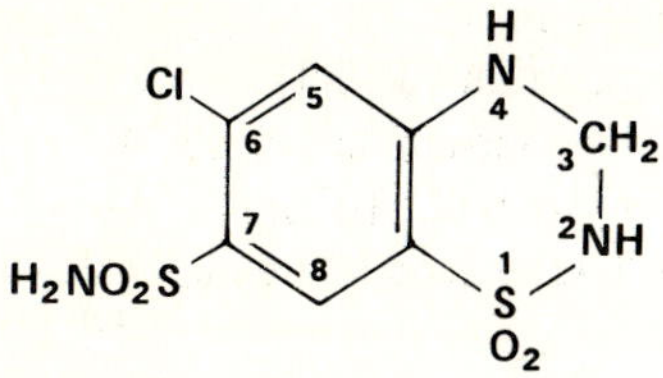

(A) Osmotic diuretics
(B) Mercurial diuretics
(C) Thiazide diuretics
(D) Carbonic anhydrase inhibitors
(E) Aldosterone antagonists

407. The LEAST distortion in the composition of extracellular fluid is caused by which of the following diuretics?

(A) Ethacrynic acid (Edecrin)
(B) Furosemide (Lasix)
(C) Hydrochlorothiazide (Hydrodiuril)
(D) Acetazolamide (Diamox)
(E) Triamterene (Dyrenium)

408. The mechanism responsible for the diuretic activity of vasopressin (Pitressin) is the

(A) activation of adenylate cyclase
(B) inhibition of prostaglandin synthesis
(C) inhibition of Na^{+}-K^{+} ATPase
(D) inhibition of carbonic anhydrase
(E) stimulation of calmodulin

409. Hyperkalemia is a contraindication to the use of which of the following drugs?

(A) Acetazolamide (Diamox)
(B) Chlorothiazide (Diuril)
(C) Ethacrynic acid (Edecrin)
(D) Furosemide (Lasix)
(E) Spironolactone (Aldactone)

410. The administration of ammonium chloride, which produces a mild metabolic acidosis, would potentiate the diuretic action of

(A) chlorothiazide (Diuril)
(B) ethacrynic acid (Edecrin)
(C) furosemide (Lasix)
(D) mercaptomerin (Thiomerin)
(E) spironolactone (Aldactone)

411. The maximum phosphaturia for any given degree of natriuresis is caused by which of the following diuretics?

(A) Ethacrynic acid (Edecrin)
(B) Furosemide (Lasix)
(C) Hydrochlorothiazide (Hydrodiuril)
(D) Acetazolamide (Diamox)
(E) Mercaptomerin (Thiomerin)

412. Acute uric acid nephropathy, which is characterized by the acute overproduction of uric acid and by extreme hyperuricemia, can best be prevented with

(A) vasopressin (ADH, Pitressin)
(B) cyclophosphamide (Cytoxan)
(C) allopurinol (Zyloprim)
(D) mercaptomerin (Thiomerin)
(E) sodium chloride

413. Mannitol, an osmotic diuretic, may be useful in all the following procedures EXCEPT

(A) treatment of elevated cerebrospinal fluid pressure
(B) treatment of elevated intraocular pressure
(C) treatment of pulmonary edema with congestive heart failure
(D) diagnostic evaluation of acute oliguria
(E) prophylaxis of acute renal failure

414. Ototoxicity is a rare but serious manifestation of

(A) mannitol
(B) ethacrynic acid (Edecrin)
(C) spironolactone (Aldactone)
(D) triamterene (Dyrenium)
(E) desmopressin acetate

415. Inhibition of dihydrofolate reductase is caused by which of the following diuretics?

(A) Mannitol
(B) Glycerin (Glycol)
(C) Acetazolamide (Diamox)
(D) Furosemide (Lasix)
(E) Triamterene (Dyrenium)

416. Very small amounts of vasopressin injected during water diuresis can cause an abrupt fall in urine flow by

(A) decreasing renal plasma flow
(B) decreasing the rate of glomerular filtration
(C) decreasing the rate of solute excretion
(D) increasing the rate of solute excretion
(E) inhibiting free water excretion

417. A hospitalized patient, who has been maintained on parenteral alimentation for three weeks, develops weakness, tremors, agitation, and finally coma. The most likely fluid and electrolyte disturbance is

(A) hyperkalemia
(B) dehydration
(C) hypomagnesemia
(D) acidosis
(E) alkalosis

418. The antidiuretic actions of vasopressin (Pitressin) are enhanced by which of the following drugs?

(A) Lithium carbonate (Eskalith)
(B) Indomethacin (Indocin)
(C) Methoxyflurane (Penthrane)
(D) Demeclocycline (Declomycin)
(E) Colchicine

DIRECTIONS: Each question below contains four suggested answers of which **one** or **more** is correct. Choose the answer:

A	if	**1, 2, and 3**	are correct
B	if	**1 and 3**	are correct
C	if	**2 and 4**	are correct
D	if	**4**	is correct
E	if	**1, 2, 3, and 4**	are correct

419. Vasopressin (Pitressin) is used therapeutically for

(1) increasing uterine contractility
(2) treating nephrogenic diabetes insipidus
(3) treating polyuria due to hypercalcemia
(4) treating neurohypophyseal diabetes insipidus

420. Osmotic diuretics have characteristics that include

(1) the capacity to be freely filtered at the glomerulus
(2) effectiveness as nonelectrolytic, osmotically active particles
(3) the ability to resist complete reabsorption by the renal tubule
(4) the ability to be metabolically altered to active forms

421. True statements about xanthine diuretics include which of the following?

(1) They are less potent than the mercurial diuretics
(2) They decrease the rate of glomerular filtration
(3) They increase cardiac output
(4) They cause a significant acidification of the urine

422. The principal side effects associated with administration of thiazide diuretics include

(1) hypernatremia
(2) hypokalemia
(3) hypoglycemia
(4) hyperuricemia

423. Drugs that may increase urea production and, therefore, contribute to prerenal azotemia include

(1) insulin
(2) triamterene
(3) penicillin
(4) tetracycline

424. Correct statements concerning the administration of spironolactone (Aldactone), a homolog of aldosterone, include which of the following?

(1) It is contraindicated in the presence of hyperkalemia
(2) It results in depression of pituitary ACTH production
(3) It can produce androgenic side effects
(4) It interferes with aldosterone synthesis

425. Side effects associated with high-ceiling diuretics like furosemide include

(1) impairment of lithium excretion
(2) metabolic alkalosis
(3) fluid and electrolyte imbalance
(4) untoward responses owing to repeated administration

426. Diuretics that function primarily in the ascending limb of the loop of Henle include

(1) hydrochlorothiazide (Esidrix)
(2) ethacrynic acid (Edecrin)
(3) chlorthalidone (Hygroton)
(4) furosemide (Lasix)

427. Thiazide diuretics increase the excretion of ions of

(1) potassium
(2) sodium
(3) magnesium
(4) calcium

428. The administration of furosemide (Lasix) or ethacrynic acid (Edecrin) results in an increased excretion of which of the following cations?

(1) Potassium
(2) Sodium
(3) Magnesium
(4) Calcium

429. Potassium excess, due to either inadequate renal excretion or extensive tissue breakdown, can be treated by administration of

(1) ammonium chloride
(2) a cation-exchange resin
(3) a thiazide diuretic
(4) calcium gluconate

430. Thiazide diuretics are clinically useful in the treatment of

(1) edema due to chronic cardiac decompensation
(2) acute renal failure secondary to transient hypotension
(3) hypertensive disease with or without overt edema
(4) glaucoma, by reducing intraocular pressure

431. Antidiuretic hormone (ADH), chlorothiazide, and other thiazide diuretics are used in the treatment of diabetes insipidus. How does the effect of thiazides differ from that of ADH in patients who have diabetes insipidus?

(1) Thiazides are effective in both nephrogenic and neurohypophyseal diabetes insipidus; ADH is not
(2) Thiazides produce a smaller volume of urine than does ADH
(3) ADH induces negative free water clearance; thiazides rarely do
(4) ADH induces potassium depletion; thiazides do not

432. Diuretics that function primarily in the distal nephron include

(1) hydrochlorothiazide (Hydrodiuril)
(2) ethacrynic acid (Edecrin)
(3) chlorthalidone (Hygroton)
(4) furosemide (Lasix)

SUMMARY OF DIRECTIONS

A	B	C	D	E
1, 2, 3 only	1, 3 only	2, 4 only	4 only	All are correct

433. True statements concerning the use of ammonium chloride as a diuretic agent include which of the following?

(1) It has a transitory effect
(2) It produces considerable gastric irritation
(3) Its ammonium portion is converted to urea, leaving an excess of chloride and causing metabolic acidosis that in turn produces diuresis
(4) It produces diuresis by functioning as an exogenous source of ammonium, resulting in decreased renal production of ammonia and in preferential excretion of sodium

434. Diuretics that are "potassium sparing" include

(1) chlorothiazide (Diuril)
(2) ethacrynic acid (Edecrin)
(3) furosemide (Lasix)
(4) triamterene (Dyrenium)

435. Increased urinary levels of Na^+ and Cl^-, no change in the urinary level of HCO_3^-, and prompt diuresis are caused by which of the following diuretic agents?

(1) Ethoxzolamide (Cardrase)
(2) Furosemide (Lasix)
(3) Acetazolamide (Diamox)
(4) Ethacrynic acid (Edecrin)

DIRECTIONS: The groups of questions below consist of lettered choices followed by several numbered items. For each numbered item select the **one** lettered choice with which it is **most** closely associated. Each lettered choice may be used once, more than once, or not at all.

Questions 436-439

For each of the following diuretic agents, choose the anatomic site in the renal nephron where the principal action of the agent occurs.

(A) Glomerulus
(B) Proximal tubule
(C) Ascending limb of the loop of Henle
(D) Distal tubule
(E) Collecting duct

436. Acetazolamide (Diamox)

437. Spironolactone (Aldactone)

438. Furosemide (Lasix)

439. Chlorothiazide (Diuril)

Questions 440-441

For each of the following pharmacologic effects, select the diuretic that is most likely to cause it.

(A) Theophylline
(B) Mercaptomerin
(C) Spironolactone
(D) Chlorothiazide
(E) Acetazolamide

440. Increases cardiac output; mild diuretic action

441. Increases bicarbonate excretion; rapidly absorbed by the gastrointestinal tract

Questions 442-444

For each of the following clinical applications or activity, select the most appropriate group of agents.

(A) Osmotic diuretics
(B) High-ceiling diuretics
(C) Thiazide (benzothiadiazide) diuretics
(D) Carbonic anhydrase inhibitors
(E) Aldosterone antagonists

442. Prophylaxis of acute renal failure in operations where hypotension is expected

443. Treatment of glaucoma

444. Has the shortest time of onset and duration of diuresis

Renal System

Answers

405. The answer is C. *(Gilman, ed 6. p 1187.)* Outdated tetracyclines have been observed to cause a form of Fanconi's syndrome, manifested by nausea, vomiting, polyuria, polydipsia, proteinuria, glycosuria, and aminoaciduria. All these findings resolve approximately one month after treatment ceases. Facial lesions similar to those seen in lupus erythematosus have also been associated with the use of outdated tetracyclines. Anhydro-4-epitetracycline, a degradation product, may be responsible for these effects.

406. The answer is C. *(Gilman, ed 6. pp 899-901.)* The structure shown in the question is hydrochlorothiazide (Esidrix) and is one of several of the thiazide (benzothiadiazide) diuretics. Halogenation of the benzothiadiazine ring at C 6 and a free sulfamyl group ($-SO_2NH_2$) at C 7 are necessary for maximal diuretic activity in this series of compounds. Benzothiadiazides, by inhibition of the reabsorption of sodium and chloride in the distal tubular portions of the nephrons, cause an increased excretion of these ions and of water. In contrast to the mercurial diuretics and to carbonic anhydrase inhibitors, benzothiadiazides can act independently of acid-base balance.

407. The answer is C. *(Gilman, ed 6. p 901.)* The thiazide diuretics, which include hydrochlorothiazide, act upon both the reabsorption of sodium and chloride in the distal segment of the tubule and the secretion of H^+. As a result of these multiple sites of actions, the thiazide diuretics produce a smaller alteration in the composition of the extracellular fluid than other classes of diuretics. This is a characteristic that makes the thiazides desirable in the chronic management of edema associated with congestive heart failure.

408. The answer is A. *(Gilman, ed 6. p 921.)* Vasopressin, or antidiuretic hormone (ADH), acts by binding to specific ADH receptors in the basolateral surface of the cortical and medullary portions of the collecting ducts. This results in the activation of adenylate cyclase, which leads to the synthesis of cyclic adenosine 3′,5′-monophosphate (cAMP). It is believed that a cAMP-dependent protein kinase is then activated, causing an increase in membrane permeability. Prostaglandin synthesis is also stimulated by ADH, and the prostaglandins may act as negative feedback inhibitors of the action of ADH.

409. The answer is E. *(Goth, ed 10. pp 497-498.)* Spironolactone (Aldactone) is a competitive antagonist of aldosterone that blocks the reabsorption of sodium and water from the distal tubule in exchange for potassium and hydrogen ion retention. Therefore, in the presence of hyperkalemia, spironolactone is contraindicated. The administration of each of the other diuretic agents listed in the question results in increased excretion of potassium.

410. The answer is D. *(Goth, ed 10. p 499.)* The ionization and, consequently, the effectiveness of mercurial diuretics such as mercaptomerin (Thiomerin) are pH-dependent. Mild acidosis induced by administration of acidifying salts promotes effectiveness of these diuretics; in conditions associated with alkalosis, the action of mercurial diuretics is antagonized. The effectiveness of the other diuretics listed in the question is relatively insensitive to acid-base balance.

411. The answer is D. *(Gilman, ed 6. p 897.)* Phosphaturia is regarded as a parameter of diuretic-induced inhibition of the reabsorption of sodium in the proximal tubule. Acetazolamide (Diamox) is the diuretic that causes the greatest phosphaturia for a given degree of natriuresis, because its effect is predominantly on the proximal tubule, where reabsorption of the phosphate ion is believed to occur. Acetazolamide is followed, in descending order, by thiazides, mercurials, and high-ceiling diuretics.

412. The answer is C. *(Isselbacher, ed 9. p 1335.)* Acute hyperuricemia, which often occurs in patients treated with cytotoxic drugs for treatment of neoplastic disorders, can lead to the deposition of urate crystals in the kidneys and their collecting ducts. This can produce partial or complete obstruction of the collecting ducts, renal pelvis, or ureter. Allopurinol and its primary metabolite, alloxanthine, are inhibitors of xanthine oxidase, an enzyme that catalyzes the oxidation of hypoxanthine and xanthine to uric acid. The use of allopurinol in patients at risk can markedly reduce the likelihood of developing acute uric acid nephropathy.

413. The answer is C. *(Gilman, ed 6. pp 895-896.)* Mannitol increases serum osmolarity and therefore "pulls" water out of cells, cerebrospinal fluid, and aqueous humor. This effect can be useful in the treatment of elevated intraocular or intracranial pressure. However, by expanding the intravascular volume, mannitol can exacerbate congestive heart failure. Mannitol will increase urine output if oliguria is caused by a decreased glomerular filtration rate but not if the oliguria is secondary to tubular dysfunction. Mannitol is useful in the prevention of acute renal failure as a means of maintaining an adequate flow of relatively dilute urine.

414. The answer is B. *(Gilman, ed 6. p 906.)* Transient or permanent deafness is a rare complication of ethacrynic acid therapy. Furosemide has also been reported to produce transient ototoxicity. Since non-high-ceiling diuretics appear free of this serious side effect, their use is recommended if other potentially ototoxic drugs, such as aminoglycoside antibiotics, are being administered.

415. The answer is E. *(Gilman, ed 6. p 909.)* Triamterene is an orally administered diuretic that acts to increase the excretion of sodium and chloride. It is a weak competitive inhibitor of dihydrofolate reductase in vitro. In patients with alcoholic cirrhosis, triamterene can produce megaloblastic anemia, which is presumably due both to the inhibition of dihydrofolate reductase by the drug and to the low levels of folic acid (due to limited intake) in these individuals.

416. The answer is E. *(Gilman, ed 6. pp 920-921.)* Vasopressin (antidiuretic hormone) acts on the cells of the collecting tubule of the kidney to increase resorption of water. This resorption is due to osmotic forces of the relatively hypertonic cortical portions of the kidney. Vasopressin, by increasing the permeability of the ductal epithelium, promotes the resorption of water. Glomerular filtration rate, renal plasma flow, and rate of solute excretion remain unchanged.

417. The answer is C. *(Gilman, ed 6. p 881.)* Hypomagnesemia is characterized by signs and symptoms that usually include disturbances in the nervous and muscular systems, psychotic behavior, tetany, tachycardia, and hypertension. Because few parenteral alimentation fluids contain magnesium, the clinical manifestations of hypomagnesemia are most commonly found in association with the prolonged parenteral alimentation of magnesium-free solutions.

418. The answer is B. *(Gilman, ed 6. p 922.)* Indomethacin can stimulate the release of vasopressin (antidiuretic hormone or ADH) and, thus, appears to enhance the actions of exogenously administered ADH. Other drugs, such as chlorpropamide, acetaminophen, cholinergic agonists, prostaglandins of the E series, and large doses of barbiturates also have similar effects. All the other drugs listed in the question inhibit the antidiuretic actions of ADH.

419. The answer is D (4). *(Isselbacher, ed 9. pp 1690-1691.)* Small doses of vasopressin (Pitressin) or the newer synthetic analog, desmopressin, can control polyuria and polydipsia in diabetes insipidus caused by neurohypophyseal insufficiency. Other syndromes that mimic the polyuria of vasopressin deficiency, such as nephrogenic diabetes insipidus and hypercalcemia, do not respond to vasopressin. Although vasopressin has intrinsic oxytocic activity, it remains relatively ineffective for initiating or intensifying uterine contractions.

420. The answer is A (1, 2, 3). *(Gilman, ed 6. p 894.)* A significant increase in the amount of any osmotically active solute in voided urine is usually accompanied by an increase in urine volume. Osmotic diuretics effect diuresis through this principle. The osmotic diuretics (such as mannitol) are nonelectrolytes that are freely filtered at the glomerulus, undergo limited resorption by the renal tubules, and—by inhibiting the transport of sodium in the proximal tubule—increase the quantity of salt supplied to the distal tubule. In addition, these diuretics resist alteration by metabolic processes.

421. The answer is B (1, 3). *(Gilman, ed 6. pp 596, 910.)* The overall potency of xanthines as diuretics is very much less than that of the mercurial diuretics or chlorothiazide. The xanthines have a combined effect on renal hemodynamics, producing increased glomerular filtration, and on tubular resorptive processes. In addition, these compounds increase cardiac output. Xanthine diuresis, which has a pattern of excretion similar to that produced by the thiazides, does not influence urinary acidification.

422. The answer is C (2, 4). *(Gilman, ed 6. pp 901-902.)* Thiazide-induced diuresis is associated with several adverse reactions, principally hypokalemia and hyperuricemia. In the renal tubules, thiazides such as chlorothiazide (Diuril) cause an increased excretion of sodium and chloride ions, and the natriuresis leads to a loss of potassium and bicarbonate ions. The hypokalemia may be corrected by administration of potassium chloride or by the administration of a preparation containing a thiazide and triamterene. The latter inhibits the sodium-potassium exchange in the distal tubule and prevents excessive loss of potassium, hydrogen, and chloride ions. Hyperuricemia may result from the competition between thiazide and uric acid for the same secretory path. Thiazide therapy may induce hyperglycemia and may exacerbate preexisting diabetes mellitus, probably by inhibition of pancreatic insulin production. Prudent management of patients receiving thiazides should include periodic evaluations for signs of hyponatremia, hypochloremic alkalosis, and hypokalemia.

423. The answer is D (4). *(Gilman, ed 6. pp 909, 1187-1188.)* Tetracycline exerts an antianabolic effect by blocking the entry of aminoacyl-transfer RNA to the adenine site; thus, the polypeptide chain cannot become elongated, protein synthesis is inhibited, and urea production is increased. Triamterine (Dyrenium) does not increase uric acid production and, unlike other diuretics, does not cause retention of uric acid.

424. The answer is B (1, 3). *(Gilman, ed 6. pp 907-908.)* Spironolactone is contraindicated in the presence of hyperkalemia, since this aldosterone antagonist may cause further elevation of plasma potassium concentrations. It does not appear to depress adrenal or pituitary function. Androgenic side effects of the drug can include hirsutism, irregular menses, and deepening of the voice. Spironolactone displaces aldosterone from receptor sites that are responsible for sodium resorption; it does not interfere with the synthesis of aldosterone.

425. The answer is A (1, 2, 3). *(Gilman, ed 6. p 906.)* Furosemide and ethacrynic acid, the high-ceiling diuretics available in the United States, are cleared by the kidney with such celerity that even high doses repeatedly administered do not result in significant accumulation. Chronic administration of these agents, however, may lead to alkalosis with hyponatremia in association with rapid removal of edema fluid. Other toxic manifestations of high-ceiling diuretics include gastrointestinal symptoms, interstitial nephritis, acute hypoglycemia, and infrequent, but serious, ototoxicity.

426. The answer is C (2, 4). *(Gilman, ed 6. pp 901, 903.)* Ethacrynic acid (Edecrin) and furosemide (Lasix) are "high-ceiling" diuretics that function primarily in the ascending limb of the loop of Henle by inhibiting the resorption of sodium and chloride ions. Thiazide, or benzothiadiazide, diuretics inhibit sodium and chloride resorption primarily in the distal portion of the nephron. These diuretics include hydrochlorothiazide (Esidrix) and chlorthalidone (Hygroton).

427. The answer is A (1, 2, 3). *(Gilman, ed 6. pp 899-902.)* Thiazide diuretics enhance the excretion of sodium, potassium, and magnesium ions. The excretion of calcium is unaffected by thiazide diuretics because distal segment resorption of this cation is not blocked by benzothiadiazides. Potassium ion excretion at the distal nephron is actively promoted by these diuretics.

428. The answer is E (all). *(Gilman, ed 6. pp 903-904.)* Furosemide (Lasix) and ethacrynic acid (Edecrin) produce a rapidity and a degree of diuresis exceeding that caused by other agents. They act by inhibiting the resorption of sodium and chloride ions in the ascending portion of Henle's loop and, by increasing the rate of flow in the distal tubules, promoting the excretion of potassium. Magnesium and calcium ions also are excreted in increased quantities.

429. The answer is C (2, 4). *(Gilman, ed 6. p 879.)* Potassium excess is best treated by cation-exchange resins given by mouth or in the form of a retention enema. If this treatment fails, either peritoneal dialysis or hemodialysis should be employed. To overcome toxic cardiac effects, which may lead to fatal arrhythmias or arrest, transient redistribution of potassium can be achieved by the intravenous administration of calcium gluconate.

430. The answer is B (1, 3). *(Gilman, ed 6. pp 901-902.)* Thiazides are most useful as diuretic agents in the management of edema due to chronic cardiac decompensation. In the treatment of hypertensive disease, even without obvious edema, thiazides exert a hypotensive action that has proved beneficial. In patients with moderate renal or hepatic insufficiency, however, these agents may aggravate the disorder by promoting fluid depletion and electrolyte imbalance. Less common uses of thiazide diuretics include the treatment of diabetes insipidus and hypercalciuria. The carbonic anhydrase inhibitor acetazolamide (Diamox), by inhibiting the secretion of aqueous humor, has the property of decreasing intraocular pressure—an effect of value for patients who have glaucoma.

431. The answer is A (1, 2, 3). *(Gilman, ed 6. pp 901, 920, 925.)* Antidiuretic hormone (ADH) is ineffective in the treatment of nephrogenic diabetes insipidus, whereas thiazides are useful in both nephrogenic and neurohypophyseal forms of the disease. ADH acts by inhibiting free water excretion; thiazides presumably act by a natriuretic effect. Thiazides result in a smaller volume of more nearly isotonic urine than does ADH in the treatment of neurohypophyseal diabetes insipidus. One of the most frequent untoward effects of the thiazides is potassium depletion.

432. The answer is B (1, 3). *(Gilman, ed 6. pp 901, 904.)* Benzothiadiazide diuretics—such as hydrochlorothiazide (Hydrodiuril), chlorthalidone (Hygroton), and other analogs of the parent structure—function primarily in the distal nephron by inhibiting resorption of sodium and chloride. The site of their action has been determined by studies utilizing stop-flow analysis, micropuncture, and interpretation of free-water production. The high-ceiling diuretics ethacrynic acid (Edecrin) and furosemide (Lasix) inhibit salt and water resorption in the ascending limb of the loop of Henle.

433. The answer is A (1, 2, 3). *(Goth, ed 10. p 499.)* Ammonium salts produce metabolic acidosis because the ammonium portion is converted to urea by the liver, resulting in an excess of chloride. The kidney responds to the metabolic acidosis by increasing production of ammonia from glutamine and other amino acids. There is, however, a delay before the kidney can produce enough ammonia to deal with the excess chloride; in the meantime, sodium is excreted while the excess chloride produces a diuretic effect. Acid-forming salts are of extremely limited value as primary diuretic agents.

434. The answer is D (4). *(Gilman, ed 6. pp 901-904, 908-909.)* Pharmacologically, ethacrynic acid (Edecrin) and furosemide (Lasix) cause potassium loss and impaired glucose tolerance. Triamterene (Dyrenium) acts as a diuretic by inhibiting resorption of sodium in exchange for potassium and hydrogen at the site in the distal tubule that is influenced by aldosterone and other mineralocorticoids. The mechanism of action of triamterene is by a direct effect on the renal tubule (not by acting as a competitor for aldosterone) and proceeds regardless of the rate of aldosterone secretion. Triamterene, which has been administered as the sole agent for producing diuresis, is most useful as an adjunct with hydrochlorothiazide in order to promote the conservation of potassium.

435. The answer is C (2, 4). *(Gilman, ed 6. pp 903-904.)* Ethoxzolamide (Cardrase) and acetazolamide (Diamox) are carbonic anhydrase inhibitors that cause increased urinary levels of Na^+, K^+, and HCO_3^-, no change in Cl^-, and decreased NH_4^+. Furosemide (Lasix) and ethacrynic acid (Edecrin) inhibit electrolyte resorption from the ascending limb of the loop of Henle, resulting in excretion of large amounts of sodium and chloride. The diuretic response to these two drugs is not significantly altered by changes in acid-base balance, and the urinary excretion of bicarbonate remains essentially unchanged.

436-439. The answers are: 436-B, 437-D, 438-C, 439-D. *(Gilman, ed 6. pp 897, 901, 903, 907.)* Acetazolamide (Diamox), a carbonic anhydrase inhibitor, until recently was thought to exert its action by inhibition of H^+ secretion by the distal tubule. Interpretation of the results of studies of free-water production and of studies in which micropuncture methods were used has provided a basis for believing that these diuretics exert a far greater effect on the proximal tubule and little if any effect on the ascending limb.

Spironolactone (Aldactone) is an aldosterone antagonist that is thought to displace aldosterone from the receptor sites responsible for sodium resorption in the distal tubule.

Furosemide (Lasix) is pharmacologically almost identical in its action with ethacrynic acid (Edecrin). They both exhibit a prompt onset of action, an independence from acid-base balance, and inhibition of sodium and chloride resorption in the ascending limb of the loop of Henle.

Chlorothiazide (Diuril), like other thiazides, inhibits the resorption of sodium and chloride in the distal tubule.

440-441. The answers are: 440-A, 441-E. *(Gilman, ed 6. pp 596, 897-898, 910.)* The naturally occurring xanthines theophylline, theobromine, and caffeine produce diuresis by increasing renal plasma flow and glomerular filtration rate. Considered to directly act on the renal tubule, they produce increased sodium and chloride excretion but no significant change in urinary pH. Xanthines have mild diuretic properties and, lacking the efficacy of other diuretics, now have limited clinical use. By stimulating the myocardium, xanthines increase the cardiac output by positive inotropic and chronotropic actions.

Acetazolamide, an inhibitor of carbonic anhydrase, increases bicarbonate excretion and suppresses the resorption of CO_2 from the glomerular filtrate. Peak plasma concentrations of acetazolamide appear within about two hours after oral administration.

442-444. The answers are: 442-A, 443-D, 444-B. *(Gilman, ed 6. pp 113, 895, 897-898, 904. Goth, ed 10, p 491.)* The maintenance of an adequate flow of relatively dilute urine is probably the most important factor in avoiding nephrotoxicity in the presence of an acutely reduced filtration rate or acute changes in tubular permeability. Osmotic diuretics exert an osmotic effect within the tubular fluid, inhibit water resorption, and maintain urine flow within reasonably normal limits. For surgical procedures in which hypotension is expected, mannitol is more effective than saline solution in maintaining adequate glomerular filtration.

The oral or parenteral administration of acetazolamide (Diamox), a carbonic anhydrase inhibitor, reduces intraocular pressure in patients who have glaucoma by reducing the rate of aqueous humor formation. Carbonic anhydrase is believed to play a part in aqueous humor secretion. Acetazolamide is a sulfonamide derivative that has been studied most often for its uses as a diuretic and a carbonic anhydrase inhibitor. The ability of acetazolamide to inhibit the activity of carbonic anhydrase appears to be related to its free $-SO_2NH_2$ group, which is a constituent of all carbonic anhydrase inhibitors.

The high-ceiling diuretics, such as ethacrynic acid (Edecrin) or furosemide (Lasix), are readily absorbed from the gastrointestinal tract and demonstrate a very rapid onset of action. In general their actions are independent of acid-base balance changes, but their duration of action is brief.

Endocrine System

DIRECTIONS: Each question below contains five suggested answers. Choose the **one best** response to each question.

445. Therapy with gonadotropins may result in

(A) amenorrhea
(B) galactorrhea
(C) ovarian hyperstimulation
(D) thyroid gland stimulation
(E) cryptorchism

446. Growth hormone replacement therapy is not useful after a bone age of 14 years because

(A) the epiphyses of the long bones are closed
(B) somatomedins are not formed after puberty
(C) the effect of growth hormone is opposed by testosterone
(D) somatostatin secretion is very high
(E) calcium resorption will be enhanced

447. A patient with diarrhea, nausea, dermatitis, and psychic disturbances is probably deficient in which of the following vitamins?

(A) Pyridoxine
(B) Thiamine
(C) Pantothenic acid
(D) Niacin
(E) Ascorbic acid

448. Ascorbic acid is an essential vitamin because it is

(A) necessary for CO_2 fixation
(B) required for conversion of proline to hydroxyproline
(C) a precursor for coenzyme A
(D) a precursor for NADP
(E) a precursor for flavin mononucleotide

449. In normal children and adults, the blood level of growth hormone rises sharply at which of the following times of day?

(A) Immediately after awakening in the morning
(B) Immediately after breakfast
(C) In the middle of the afternoon
(D) In the early evening
(E) In the early part of sleep

450. A substance that enhances the probability of ovulation by blocking the inhibitory effect of estrogens and thus stimulating the release of gonadotropin from the pituitary is

(A) androstenedione
(B) clomiphene (Clomid)
(C) diethylstilbestrol
(D) ethinyl estradiol
(E) progesterone

451. The hormone useful in treating Paget's disease of bone is

(A) aldosterone
(B) cortisol
(C) calcitonin
(D) parathyroid hormone
(E) thyroxine

452. The requirement for thiamine is greatest under which of the following conditions?

(A) Stressful procedures
(B) Consumption of megadoses of vitamin C
(C) High fat diet
(D) High protein diet
(E) High carbohydrate diet

453. The diagnostic agent useful in identifying both hypo- and hyperthyroidism is

(A) thyroxine
(B) triiodothyronine
(C) thyroid-stimulating hormone
(D) thyrotropin-releasing hormone
(E) long-acting thyroid stimulator

454. A patient becomes markedly tetanic following a recent thyroidectomy. This symptom can be **rapidly** reversed by the administration of

(A) vitamin D
(B) calcitonin
(C) parathyroid hormone
(D) thyroid extract
(E) calcium gluconate

455. The antithyroid action of propylthiouracil is thought to involve which of the following mechanisms?

(A) Blocking the enzymatic oxidation of iodide
(B) Preventing the uptake of iodide
(C) Preventing the synthesis of thyroglobulin
(D) Inhibiting the release of thyroid-stimulating hormone
(E) Blocking the release of thyroxine

456. The steroid used in standard pituitary-adrenal suppression tests is

(A) cortisone
(B) hydrocortisone
(C) dexamethasone
(D) fludrocortisone (Flurinef)
(E) androstenedione

457. Steroid compounds include all the following EXCEPT

(A) androsterone
(B) clomiphene (Clomid)
(C) ethynodiol diacetate (Demulen)
(D) etiocholanolone
(E) norethindrone

458. Metyrapone is useful in testing the endocrine functioning of the

(A) α cells of pancreatic islets
(B) β cells of pancreatic islets
(C) neurohypophysis
(D) pituitary-adrenal axis
(E) Leydig cells of testes

459. The steroid having the greatest anti-inflammatory potency is which of the following?

(A) Cortisone
(B) Hydrocortisone
(C) Prednisone
(D) Dexamethasone
(E) Triamcinolone

460. Protamine is added to insulin in order to

(A) speed the absorption of insulin from the injection site by increasing insulin solubility
(B) speed the absorption of insulin by increasing the local blood flow
(C) slow the absorption of insulin by constricting blood vessels
(D) slow the absorption of insulin by promoting insulin binding to tissue proteins
(E) slow the absorption of insulin by forming a relatively insoluble complex

461. Insulin accelerates glucose transport across membranes in

(A) brain tissue
(B) hepatic tissue
(C) heart muscle
(D) leukocytes
(E) erythrocytes

462. The insulin preparation having the longest duration of action is which of the following?

(A) Insulin injection (regular insulin)
(B) Prompt insulin zinc suspension (Semilente)
(C) Isophane insulin suspension, or NPH insulin
(D) Insulin zinc suspension (Lente)
(E) Protamine zinc insulin suspension (PZI)

463. Bromocriptine (Parlodel) is used to treat some cases of infertility because it

(A) stimulates release of gonadotropin-releasing hormone
(B) stimulates the ovary directly
(C) is an estrogen antagonist that enhances gonadotropin release
(D) inhibits prolactin release
(E) increases the synthesis of follicle-stimulating hormone

464. Tamoxifen is used to treat some breast cancers because of its ability to

(A) utilize its androgenic properties in retarding tumor growth
(B) prevent estrogen synthesis by the ovary
(C) enhance glucocorticoid treatment
(D) act as an estrogen antagonist
(E) act as a potent progestin

465. The general structure for thyroid hormones is shown below. In order for this structure to acquire significant hormone activity, all the following modifications must take place EXCEPT that

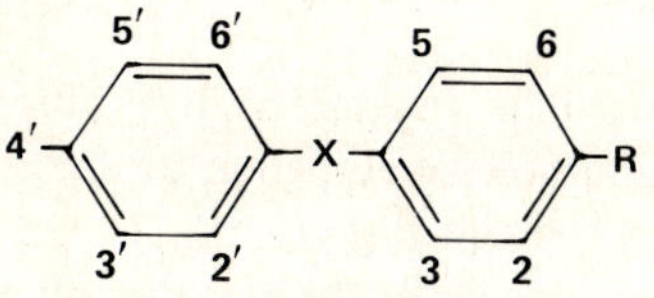

(A) the connection between the two aromatic rings should be by ether, thioether, or methylene linkage
(B) the R side chain on carbon 1 should be aliphatic and contain a carboxyl group
(C) halogenation or methylation is necessary at positions 3 and 5
(D) a hydroxyl group should be on position 3′
(E) position 4′ should have a hydroxyl group or a group capable of being metabolically converted to hydroxyl

DIRECTIONS: Each question below contains four suggested answers of which **one** or **more** is correct. Choose the answer:

A	if	1, 2, and 3	are correct
B	if	1 and 3	are correct
C	if	2 and 4	are correct
D	if	4	is correct
E	if	1, 2, 3, and 4	are correct

466. Endogenous vasopressin release is inhibited by which of the following drugs?

(1) Phenytoin
(2) Nicotine
(3) Ethanol
(4) Morphine

467. True statements about oxytocin include which of the following?

(1) It is approved for use in elective induction of labor
(2) It causes postpartum hemorrhage
(3) It causes a large increase in blood pressure
(4) It should be administered intravenously to induce labor

468. Absence of aldosterone in a patient who has Addison's disease is associated with

(1) hypernatremia
(2) cellular hydration
(3) hypokalemia
(4) hypovolemia

469. Actions that usually will cause an increase in the serum level of growth hormone in a normal person include

(1) fasting for more than 48 hours
(2) an intravenous infusion of arginine
(3) administration of insulin to induce hypoglycemia
(4) ingestion of a glucose solution

470. True statements concerning the pharmacologic properties of thyroxine (T_4) and triiodothyronine (T_3) in humans include which of the following?

(1) T_4 is more potent than T_3
(2) T_4 has a longer half-life than T_3
(3) Only T_4 can be administered orally
(4) T_4 has a greater affinity for thyroxine-binding prealbumin than T_3

Questions 471-472

A 39-year-old, gravida 3, para 3, woman is admitted to a gynecology clinic for evaluation of vaginal pruritis. She had not been examined by a physician for six years, since the birth of her youngest child. She has no pubic or axillary hair; her skin is cold, dry, thin, soft, and finely wrinkled; she appears moderately anemic, and exhibits vitiligo on her hands. She has experienced cold sensitivity, a deepening of her voice, recurrent dermal infections, and amenorrhea since the birth of her last child.

471. The findings, symptoms, and history described above are consistent with which of the following disorders?

(1) Sheehan's syndrome
(2) Addisonian syndrome
(3) Myxedema
(4) Craniopharyngioma

472. The patient described above can expect her appearance and general health to return to normal if she is given

(1) thyroid extract
(2) prednisone
(3) diethylstilbestrol
(4) insulin

473. A deficiency in vitamin A results in which of the following defects?

(1) Enhanced susceptibility to carcinogens
(2) Night blindness
(3) Keratomalacia
(4) Cancellous bone formation

474. Pseudohermaphroditism has been shown to be caused by which of the following conditions?

(1) A deficiency in 5α-reductase activity
(2) An increased conversion of testosterone to estrogen
(3) Lack of a dihydrotestosterone receptor
(4) Competition of progesterone with the testosterone receptor

475. The intravenous injection of 0.1 unit of regular insulin per kilogram of body weight in a normal individual will usually cause significantly increased plasma levels of

(1) cortisol
(2) triamcinolone
(3) growth hormone
(4) glucose

476. The "minipill" containing only a progestin, rather than a combined estrogen-progestin oral contraceptive, was developed because

(1) progestin alone is a more effective contraceptive agent than the two combined
(2) progestin alone results in a more regular menstrual cycle
(3) the combination of estrogen and progestin induces endometriosis
(4) progestin alone is thought to be less likely to induce cardiovascular disorders

477. Parathyroid hormone has which of the following physiologic effects?

(1) Increased mobilization of calcium from bone
(2) Decreased active absorption of calcium from the small intestine
(3) Increased resorption of phosphate from bone
(4) Decreased renal tubular reabsorption of calcium

478. Vigorous exercise by a well-controlled, insulin-dependent diabetic person can promote

(1) glycosuria
(2) an increased insulin requirement
(3) hyperglycemia
(4) glucose transport into muscle cells

479. Physical characteristics that are typical of an adult eunuch include which of the following?

(1) Facies of a child
(2) Short stature
(3) High-pitched voice
(4) Normal axillary and pubic hair

SUMMARY OF DIRECTIONS

A	B	C	D	E
1, 2, 3 only	1, 3 only	2, 4 only	4 only	All are correct

480. The serum of women contains which of the following steroid hormones?

(1) Estrone
(2) Progesterone
(3) Estradiol
(4) Testosterone

481. In nephrectomized animals, active forms of vitamin D include

(1) cholecalciferol
(2) cod liver oil
(3) ergocalciferol
(4) dihydrotachysterol

482. Glucocorticoids endogenously released from the adrenal cortex include

(1) cortisol
(2) aldosterone
(3) corticosterone
(4) triamcinolone

483. Bilateral adrenalectomy can be expected to result in

(1) hypotension
(2) hypoglycemia
(3) hyperkalemia
(4) hypernatremia

484. Steroids that are synthesized in the adrenal gland include which of the following?

(1) Pregnenolone
(2) Progesterone
(3) Corticosterone
(4) 9α-Fluorocortisol

485. The administration of corticosteroids can be beneficial in the treatment of

(1) severe bronchial asthma
(2) chronic ulcerative colitis
(3) anterior pituitary insufficiency
(4) pheochromocytoma

486. Manifestations of hyperprolactinemia include

(1) amenorrhea
(2) galactorrhea
(3) impotency
(4) hypothyroidism

487. Insulin secretion in normal humans can be promoted by administration of which of the following substances?

(1) Glucagon
(2) Growth hormone
(3) Acetohexamide (Dymelor)
(4) Somatostatin

488. Insulin deficiency enhances which of the following conversions?

(1) Protein to glucose
(2) Fat depots to plasma free fatty acids
(3) Protein to urinary ammonia and urea
(4) Glucose to glycogen

489. Metabolic actions promoted by glucagon include

(1) glycogenolysis
(2) fat synthesis
B (3) gluconeogenesis
(4) peripheral glucose utilization

DIRECTIONS: The groups of questions below consist of lettered choices followed by several numbered items. For each numbered item select the **one** lettered choice with which it is **most** closely associated. Each lettered choice may be used once, more than once, or not at all.

Questions 490-493

Match the following.

(A) Triiodothyronine
(B) Bromocriptine (Parlodel)
(C) Clomiphene (Clomid)
(D) Dexamethasone
(E) Haloperidol (Haldol)

490. Stimulates release of gonadotropins

491. Stimulates prolactin release

492. Suppresses stimulation of hormone release by thyrotropin-releasing hormone (TRH)

493. Inhibits growth hormone release in some acromegalic patients

Questions 494-496

For each of the following drugs, choose the vitamin, metabolic cofactor, or precursor of which it is a structural analog.

(A) *p*-Aminobenzoic acid
(B) Calciferol
(C) Folic acid
(D) Nicotinamide
(E) Vitamin K

494. Methotrexate

495. Sulfanilamide

496. Warfarin

Questions 497-500

For each inhibitory effect on thyroid hormone synthesis listed below, select the agent that causes it.

(A) Sodium thiocyanate
(B) Methimazole (Tapazole)
(C) Triiodothyronine
(D) Radioactive iodine
(E) Iodide

497. Inhibits, by acting as a competitor, the accumulation of iodide in thyroid follicular cells

498. Inhibits the peroxidase-catalyzed oxidation of iodide and thus interferes with the incorporation of iodide into an organic structure

499. Inhibits the peroxidase-catalyzed coupling of iodotyrosines to form iodothyronines

500. Inhibits the secretion of hormone

Endocrine System

Answers

445. The answer is C. *(Gilman, ed 6. pp 1386-1387.)* Menotropins, derived from the urine of postmenopausal women, and chorionic gonadotropin, derived from the urine of pregnant women, are used to treat infertility. Ovarian hyperstimulation may occur and result in pain and bleeding. The incidence of multiple births is also higher than normal, occurring in 20% of gonadotropin-induced pregnancies.

446. The answer is A. *(Gilman, ed 6. p 1378.)* Growth hormone is used successfully to treat a deficiency of the hormone but is most effective when patients are treated early. If the patient has gone through puberty, the epiphyses of the long bones are closed, a process stimulated by testosterone, and further growth will be limited. Growth hormone exerts many of its effects by stimulating the release of somatomedins.

447. The answer is D. *(Gilman, ed 6. p 1568.)* Niacin, or nicotinic acid, is converted into NAD and NADP, which are necessary for a variety of oxidation-reduction enzyme reactions. Tryptophan may be used instead of nicotinic acid to synthesize the coenzymes. A deficiency of niacin causes pellagra, characterized by diarrhea and gastrointestinal disturbances, dermatitis, and dementia.

448. The answer is B. *(Gilman, ed 6. pp 1577-1579.)* Ascorbic acid, or vitamin C, is involved in a number of oxidative reactions, including the conversion of proline to hydroxyproline in the synthesis of collagen. Lack of ascorbic acid produces scurvy, with bleeding gums and poor wound healing, probably reflecting poor collagen synthesis. Megadoses of vitamin C can cause kidney stone formation.

449. The answer is E. *(Martin, p 153.)* The blood level of growth hormone (GH) rises sharply about one hour after the beginning of sleep. This initial rise in GH is not just a reflection of circadian rhythm—the peak secretion occurs within two hours of the start of sleep. In an individual who is kept awake all night or who is permitted to nap frequently but only briefly each time, the rise in concentration of growth hormone will be postponed until the subject finally enters sleep.

450. The answer is B. *(Gilman, ed 6. p 1433.)* Clomiphene (Clomid) is an effective fertility drug that can lead to multiple pregnancies. Clomiphene has been termed an antiestrogen because its stimulant effect on the secretion of pituitary gonadotropins is thought to be the consequence of its blocking the inhibitory effect of estrogens on gonadotropin secretion. Side effects of this drug can include ovarian enlargement and cysts, and premature menopausal symptoms.

451. The answer is C. *(Gilman, ed 6. p 1538.)* Calcitonin is useful in the therapy of Paget's disease of bone (osteitis deformans). Calcitonin therapy reduces urinary hydroxyproline excretion and serum alkaline phosphatase activity and provides some symptomatic relief. Presumably these effects result from the ability of calcitonin to inhibit bone resorption. Side effects of long-term therapy with this hormone can include nausea, edema of the hands, and urticaria. The apperance of neutralizing antibodies may explain the development of resistance to treatment.

452. The answer is E. *(Gilman, ed 6. pp 1560-1563.)* Thiamine pyrophosphate is formed from thiamine and acts as a coenzyme in the decarboxylation of α-ketoglutarate and pyruvate, as well as the hexose monophosphate shunt. Therefore, it is an important part of carbohydrate metabolism. Patients who are being maintained on dextrose need extra amounts of the vitamin. Under normal circumstances, 1 mg per day is recommended.

453. The answer is D. *(Martin, pp 221-222.)* Thyrotropin-releasing hormone (TRH) stimulates the pituitary gland to release thyroid-stimulating hormone (TSH). The effect of TRH is antagonized by small increases in thyroid hormone. Consequently, the increment in TSH in response to TRH injection is abnormally small in the presence of hyperthyroidism. Similarly, the increment in TSH is abnormally large in most patients with hypothyroidism. Even minor changes in thyroid hormone blood levels may elicit these changes.

454. The answer is E. *(Gilman, ed 6. pp 1528, 1534.)* Administration of intravenous calcium gluconate would immediately correct the tetany that might occur in a patient in whom a thyroidectomy was recently performed. Parathyroid hormone would act more slowly but could be given for its future stabilizing effect. Long-term control of a patient after a thyroidectomy can be obtained with vitamin D and dietary therapy. Calcitonin is a hypocalcemic antagonist of parathyroid hormone.

455. The answer is A. *(Gilman, ed 6. pp 1409-1410.)* The formation of thyroxine is inhibited by antithyroid agents such as propylthiouracil, which probably interferes with the peroxidase-mediated oxidation of iodide in the ring iodination of tyrosine. The utilization of hydrogen peroxide in the oxidation of iodide by the enzyme is a key reaction that some investigators suspect is inhibited by propylthiouracil. That propylthiouracil inhibits the synthesis of thyroid hormones and does not inactivate colloid stores of or circulating levels of thyroxine and triiodothyronine is generally accepted.

456. The answer is C. *(Craig, p 823.)* Dexamethasone is a long-acting glucocorticoid that shuts off the secretion of ACTH by the anterior pituitary and, as a result, decreases synthesis of steroids by the adrenals. Thus, dexamethasone leads to decreased 17-hydroxycorticosteroid excretion in the urine. Because of the great potency of dexamethasone, it can be used in such small quantities that its presence in the urine does not interfere with the measurement of endogenous steroid excretion.

457. The answer is B. *(Gilman, ed 6. pp 1432-1433.)* All the compounds listed in the question are steroids, with the exception of clomiphene (Clomid), an estrogen analog that lacks the essential feature of a steroid: a hydrogenated cyclopentenophenanthrene-ring system. Clomid is a derivative of the weakly estrogenic compound chlorotrianisene. The *cis*-form has a high antiestrogenic activity that inhibits estrogenic feedback repression of gonadotropin secretion. Clomid is an effective fertility-inducing drug.

458. The answer is D. *(Gilman, ed 6. p 1492.)* Metyrapone (Metopirone), because it decreases serum levels of cortisol by inhibiting the 11β-hydroxylation of steroids in the adrenal, can be used to assess the function of the pituitary-adrenal axis. When metyrapone is administered orally or intravenously to normal persons, the adenohypophysis will secrete an increased amount of adrenocorticotropic hormone (ACTH). This will cause a normal adrenal gland to synthesize increased amounts of 17-hydroxylated steroids that can be measured in the urine. However, patients who have disease of the hypothalamico-pituitary complex are not able to respond to administration of metyrapone by producing increased amounts of ACTH; consequently, no increased levels of 17-hydroxylated steroids would be detected in the urine. Before administering the drug, the ability of the adrenal gland to respond to ACTH must be tested.

459. The answer is D. *(Craig, p 816.)* Cortisone, when first used for its anti-inflammatory effect, was associated with increased sodium retention, decreased carbohydrate tolerance, and other toxic responses. Recently, however, compounds have been produced that cause no serious effects on electrolyte balance, although the effects on carbohydrate and protein metabolism—like the promotion of gluconeogenesis—remain. Dexamethasone is the most potent of the various anti-inflammatory steroids: it is 20 times as effective as hydrocortisone and therefore requires the lowest daily dose (4 mg/ml). It has almost no sodium-retaining potency.

460. The answer is E. *(Gilman, ed 6. p 1508.)* The complex that is formed if insulin reacts with the basic protein protamine has an approximate isoelectric point of pH 7.3 and is, therefore, relatively insoluble in body fluids. When an aqueous suspension of the complex is injected subcutaneously, the slow dissolution at the injection site allows absorption of the insulin at a slow but steady rate. Protamine zinc insulin suspension, for example, is classified as a long-acting insulin preparation that has a duration of action of about 36 hours.

461. The answer is C. *(Gilman, ed 6. p 1505.)* Insulin, an anabolic hormone that controls major metabolic pathways, is not required to facilitate glucose transport across membranes of erythrocytes, leukocytes, or across membranes in the liver, brain, or renal medulla. Insulin accelerates glucose transport across membranes in cardiac, skeletal, and adipose tissues, although glucose transport is increased across muscle cell membranes during exercise even when insulin is absent. After exposure to insulin, membrane proteins undergo altered phosphorylation; however, little is known about the mechanism by which insulin facilitates the transport of glucose and other hexoses across certain membranes.

462. The answer is E. *(Gilman, ed 6. pp 1508-1509.)* Insulin injection (also known as regular or unmodified insulin) is effective for about 6 hours; prompt insulin zinc suspension (Semilente), for about 14 hours; isophane insulin suspension (also known as NPH insulin), for about 24 hours; insulin zinc suspension (Lente), for about 24 hours; and protamine zinc insulin suspension (also known as PZI), for about 36 hours. The latter, first prepared in 1936, is a complexed protein that, because of its chemical nature, dissolves slowly at the injection site to allow the insulin to be absorbed slowly and steadily. Extended Insulin Zinc Suspension, also effective for 36 hours, is a slowly dissolving insulin and zinc mixture that has no protamine.

463. The answer is D. *(Gilman, ed 6. p 1382. Martin, pp 361-363.)* High prolactin levels in the serum result in amenorrhea, for reasons that are not known. Bromocriptine inhibits prolactin secretion through its dopaminergic action and has been recently approved for use in treating infertility caused by hyperprolactinemia. High prolactin levels often result from pituitary tumors, and bromocriptine has been reported to cause these tumors to regress.

464. The answer is D. *(Gilman, ed 6. p 1304.)* Tamoxifen is an estrogen antagonist used in the treatment of breast cancer. Postmenopausal women with metastases to soft tissue and whose tumors contain an estrogen receptor are most likely to respond to this agent. Little benefit is derived from tamoxifen if the tumor does not have estrogen receptors.

465. The answer is D. *(Gilman, ed 6. p 1398.)* According to extensive research on the relationship between structure and activity of thyronine derivatives, significant thyroid hormone activity would be characteristic of the structure:

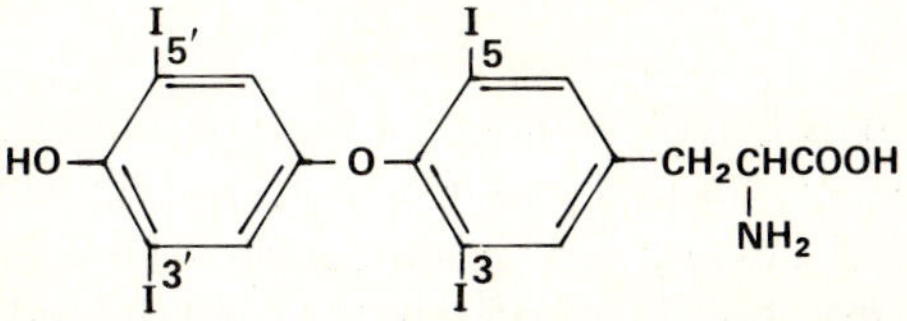

This structure is thyroxine, in which the R side chain is L-alanine, the aromatic rings are connected by an ether linkage, halogenation by iodine occurs on positions 3,5 and 3′,5′, and a hydroxyl group is attached to carbon 4′. Activity can be increased four-fold upon removing iodine from the 5′ position because 3′-monosubstituted compounds have more activity than 3′,5′-disubstituted derivatives of thyronine.

466. The answer is B (1, 3). *(Martin, p 71.)* Ethanol inhibits vasopressin release in response to changes in blood volume and to dehydration but not in response to hemorrhage or nicotine. Therefore, ethanol can provoke inappropriate water diuresis and dehydration. Phenytoin, in relatively large doses, can also suppress the release of vasopressin. Nicotine, morphine, and many general anesthetics cause vasopressin release.

467. The answer is D (4). *(Gilman, ed 6. pp 947-949.)* Oxytocin is used to induce or stimulate labor that is medically indicated; it should not be used for elective inductions. When used for inductions, it should be administered intravenously so that the rate of infusion can be controlled. If too much oxytocin is administered, a sustained tetanic contraction can result, which may rupture the uterus or cause fetal hypoxia.

468. The answer is C (2, 4). *(Gilman, ed 6. pp 1475, 1488.)* Mineralocorticoids such as aldosterone and desoxycorticosterone stimulate the renal distal tubules to increase their reabsorption of sodium ions and cause the increased loss of potassium and hydrogen ions. In the absence of aldosterone, as in Addison's disease, 98.5 percent of filtered sodium is reabsorbed (in normal persons, 99.5 percent is reabsorbed). Thus, aldosterone, considered the most potent of naturally occurring corticosteroid electrolyte-balance regulators, causes an additional 1 percent to be reabsorbed, a percentage that represents 240 mEq of ionic sodium per day. The daily loss of this quantity of sodium ions occurs in patients who have Addison's disease and is sufficiently substantial to cause hyponatremia, an increased hematocrit value due to hypovolemia and cellular hydration, and hyperkalemia—effects that lead to circulatory collapse, renal failure, and death. An acute addisonian crisis would be treated with isotonic saline (containing glucose to compensate for hypoglycemia and deficient nutrition) and with cortisol.

469. The answer is E (all). *(Gilman, ed 6. p 1377.)* Plasma levels of growth hormone (GH) in normal persons can be increased by each of the actions listed in the question. A 60-hour fast usually results in an increase of plasma GH to about 8 ng/ml (the normal level after a 12-hour fast ranges from 0 to 3 ng/ml). This elevated GH level returns rapidly to normal after a meal or ingestion of a glucose solution. In normal adults and in some normal children, GH levels can be increased to 25 to 50 ng/ml within 30 minutes after an insulin-induced hypoglycemia characterized by a decrease in the blood glucose level that is less than 50 percent of that in the fasting state. The intravenous infusion of 30 g of arginine during a period of 30 minutes usually produces an increase in GH levels in normal adults and children and is regarded as a safer provocative test of the capacity of the pituitary to secrete GH than the use of insulin. Within about 4 hours after the ingestion of a glucose solution, as used in the glucose tolerance test, GH levels usually increase. Lack, or undetectable levels, of GH does not in itself warrant a diagnosis of adenohypophyseal hypofunction. Evaluation of more than one test and of the health status of the patient is needed to identify a growth hormone deficiency due to hypofunction of the anterior pituitary.

470. The answer is C (2, 4). *(Gilman, ed 6. pp 1397, 1400-1402, 1406.)* In structure-activity studies, 3′-monosubstituted compounds such as 3,5,3′-triiodothyronine (T_3) have been shown to be about four times more potent than 3′,5′-disubstituted compounds such as thyroxine (T_4). Both T_3 and T_4 can be administered orally; the sodium salt of the latter is believed to be better absorbed after oral administration than the preparation made by the defatting and desiccation of thyroids selected from slaughtered animals. T_3, probably because it is less strongly bound to protein, has a half-life of two days or less, whereas that of T_4 is six to seven days. By the mechanism of deiodination, T_4 is converted to T_3 in the liver and kidneys, according to the conclusions of recent radioimmunoassay studies.

471. The answer is E (all). *(Gilman, ed 6. pp 1371-1372.)* The findings, symptoms, and history described in the question are typical of a patient who has hypopituitarism, whether the cause be postpartum pituitary necrosis (Sheehan's syndrome), as is likely in this case, or a pituitary tumor. Sheehan's syndrome is thought to be caused by the normally reduced blood flow to the pituitary that occurs during delivery, being accentuated by the severe circulatory collapse associated with postpartum hemorrhage. Blood flow to the anterior lobe may be so reduced that thrombosis and infarction occur. Hypothyroidism (myxedema) and hypoadrenocorticism (addisonian syndrome) are secondary to the loss of the pituitary stimulus.

472. The answer is A (1, 2, 3). *(Gilman, ed 6. pp 1371-1372.)* Thyroid extract, a corticosteroid, and a feminizing sex hormone would be sufficient therapy for the recovery of the patient described in the previous question. She would still lack growth hormone, ACTH, and other hormones—but the lack would not be detectable clinically. The woman is not insulin dependent.

473. The answer is E (all). *(Gilman, ed 6. pp 1583-1586.)* Hippocrates recommended beef liver to cure night blindness—a valid suggestion because retinal is necessary to form rhodopsin, the pigment in the eye bleached by light, and liver is a good source of vitamin A (retinol), which can form retinal. In addition to night blindness, vitamin A deficiency can cause keratomalacia and cancellous bone formation. Lack of vitamin A also enhances susceptibility to carcinogenesis in experimental animals and in humans.

474. The answer is B (1, 3). *(Gilman, ed 6. p 1453.)* Testosterone must be converted to dihydrotestosterone in order for the hormone to become active at many sites. Dihydrotestosterone binds to a cytoplasmic receptor and is transferred to the nucleus. Male pseudohermaphroditism has been caused by lack of the converting enzyme, 5α-reductase, or lack of a dihydrotestosterone receptor.

475. The answer is B (1, 3). *(Gilman, ed 6. pp 1377, 1469. Martin, pp 326-328.)* Circadian rhythm and stress are major factors that influence cortisol secretion. Stress factors such as trauma of surgery, pyrogenic infections, and hypoglycemia all can stimulate ACTH secretion and, thereby, increase plasma levels of cortisol. Insulin-induced hypoglycemia, by intravenous administration of 0.1 unit of regular insulin per kg of body weight, can be expected to increase plasma levels of cortisol by 10-20 μg/100 ml in about 90 minutes after injection in normal persons. The plasma level of growth hormone in the resting, preprandial person can be increased from the normal range of 0 to 3 ng/ml to 10 to 50 ng/ml within about 30 minutes after an insulin injection. Compared to the metyrapone test—which can be used to evaluate the feedback control mechanism regulating ACTH secretion—insulin-induced hypoglycemia generally is regarded as the more vigorous stimulus to ACTH secretion.

476. The answer is D (4). *(Gilman, ed 6. pp 1440-1444.)* The combination of estrogen and progestin is the most effective means of preventing contraception; progestin alone is less effective. Menstruation will occur with progestin alone, but it may be irregular. Estrogen is thought to cause the increased incidence of thrombophlebitis and cerebral and coronary thrombosis that is found in women taking combined oral contraceptives.

477. The answer is B (1, 3). *(Craig, pp 874-876.)* Parathyroid hormone (PTH) is synthesized by and released from the parathyroid gland; increased synthesis of PTH is a response to low serum calcium concentrations. Resorption or mobilization of calcium and phosphate from bone is increased in response to elevated PTH concentrations. Replacement of body stores of calcium is enhanced by the capacity of PTH to promote increased absorption of calcium by the small intestine. PTH also causes an increased renal tubular reabsorption of calcium and excretion of phosphate. As a consequence of these effects, the extracellular calcium concentration becomes elevated.

478. The answer is D (4). *(Gilman, ed 6. pp 1509, 1514-1515.)* Vigorous exercise promotes the transport of glucose into muscle cells and the utilization of carbohydrates in the well-controlled, insulin-dependent diabetic patient. Hypoglycemia can result, and the patient's insulin requirement will be decreased. Conversely, if the same well-controlled diabetic patient suddenly becomes sedentary, the insulin requirement probably will become increased.

479. The answer is B (1, 3). *(Gilman, ed 6. p 1452.)* An adult eunuch retains childhood facies, is abnormally tall with particularly long limbs, has a high-pitched voice because the larynx does not grow, and has sparse axillary and pubic hair. In addition, he has underdeveloped musculature, a body form mistakenly interpreted as "feminine" owing to the deposition and distribution of subcutaneous fat, child-like genitalia, and no sexual drive.

480. The answer is E (all). *(Gilman, ed 6. pp 1422, 1427, 1450-1451.)* Progesterone, synthesized from cholesterol, is converted into androstenedione through identical steps in the ovary, testis, and adrenal cortex. Androstenedione may be transformed into estrone directly or to estradiol via testosterone. Testosterone is elaborated in the testis, adrenal cortex, as well as ovary; the testosterone plasma level in women is about one tenth of that in men.

481. The answer is D (4). *(Gilman, ed 6. pp 1539-1540, 1544.)* Dihydrotachysterol, when compared to vitamin D_3, has its A ring rotated so that its 3-hydroxyl group is located in almost the same position as the 1-hydroxyl group of 1,25-dihydroxycholecalciferol. Consequently, dihydrotachysterol requires only hydroxylation at position 25 to be active. Because hydroxylation at position 1 occurs in the kidney, only dihydrotachysterol is active in a nephrectomized animal.

482. The answer is B (1, 3). *(Gilman, ed 6. p 1473.)* Cortisol and corticosterone are glucocorticoids and are endogenously released from the adrenal cortex. Aldosterone, also endogenously released from the adrenal gland, is classified as a mineralocorticoid. The terms "glucocorticoid" and "mineralocorticoid," as applied to corticosteroids, are designations that indicate the major actions of these agents: the actual biologic characteristics of corticosteroids range over a spectrum. Thus corticosterone, classed as a glucocorticoid, also has some activity as a mineralocorticoid. Triamcinolone is a synthetic steroid preparation.

483. The answer is A (1, 2, 3). *(Gilman, ed 6. pp 1474-1476, 1488.)* A person who has Addison's disease and is not receiving medical treatment, or who has had a bilateral adrenalectomy, can expect to be hypotensive and have hypoglycemia, hyponatremia, and hyperkalemia. Lethargy, anorexia, muscle weakness, hyperpigmentation, and gastrointestinal symptoms are other symptoms of adrenal insufficiency. Therapy for the chronic adrenal insufficiency that results from adrenal surgery or that is associated with Addison's disease should consist of administration of cortisone acetate, 25 to 37.5 mg/day, and usually a strong mineralocorticoid.

484. The answer is A (1, 2, 3). *(Gilman, ed 6. pp 1472, 1481-1482.)* Pregnenolone is synthesized from cholesterol in an ACTH-regulated enzymic oxidation and cleavage of the aliphatic side chain attached to C 17 of the steroid ring. Progesterone, desoxycorticosterone, corticosterone, and aldosterone are sequential products derived from the pregnenolone precursor. 9α-Fluorocortisol, or fludrocortisone (Florinef), a synthetic steroid, is among the most potent mineralocorticoids and is used frequently in patients who require partial replacement therapy for adrenocortical insufficiency in Addison's disease.

485. The answer is A (1, 2, 3). *(Gilman, ed 6. pp 1482-1483, 1488-1491.)* The administration of corticosteroids can be helpful as supplements to epinephrine in terminating an acute asthmatic attack and in treating the disabling symptoms of chronic bronchial asthma if other treatments fail. Corticosteroids are also useful in treating adrenal insufficiency secondary to anterior pituitary insufficiency. In chronic ulcerative colitis, severely ill patients who have fever, anorexia, anemia, and malnutrition can improve dramatically when given systemic steroids. Pheochromocytoma is a tumor of the adrenal medulla and is unresponsive to adrenocortical preparations. Before administering corticosteroids, physicians should consider that long-term therapy with these drugs has been associated with substantial side effects and that abrupt termination of high-dosage corticosteroids administered over a long period of time can cause severe or lethal adrenal insufficiency.

486. The answer is E (all). *(Gilman, ed 6. p 1382. Martin, p 137.)* High prolactin levels can stimulate the breast to secrete, causing galactorrhea in about 30 percent of patients with hyperprolactinemia. Amenorrhea in women and impotency in men may also result; the mechanisms by which prolactin causes these effects is not known. Hypothyroidism may be accompanied by high prolactin levels, presumably because a large amount of thyrotropin-releasing hormone, which also releases prolactin, is being released from the hypothalamus. Hyperprolactinemia can be treated with bromocriptine (Parlodel) except when caused by hypothyroidism (in this case, the treatment should be thyroid hormone).

487. The answer is A (1, 2, 3). *(Gilman, ed 6. pp 1500, 1511.)* Glucagon and growth hormone cause insulin secretion by promoting hyperglycemia. Acetohexamide, a sulfonylurea compound, degranulates β cells of the pancreatic islets, releasing insulin from patients who can still synthesize their own. Somatostatin, originally isolated from the hypothalamus, inhibits the release of growth hormone, insulin, and glucagon. Somatostatin is found in the pancreas as well as the hypothalamus.

488. The answer is A (1, 2, 3). *(Gilman, ed 6. pp 1503-1506.)* In an insulin-deficient state, there is degradation of proteins to amino acids with conversion to glucose, ammonia, and urea, all of which may be excreted. Fat depots are mobilized because the inhibitory effects of insulin on a fat-mobilizing lipase are lost. Likewise, glycogen synthetase, which is stimulated by insulin, functions at a reduced rate, thus retarding the conversion of glucose to glycogen.

489. The answer is B (1, 3). *(Gilman, ed 6. p 1518.)* Glucagon and insulin are generally regarded as mutual antagonists. Glucagon, synthesized in the pancreatic α cells, promotes glycogenolysis and gluconeogenesis; insulin, produced in the pancreatic β cells, promotes fat synthesis and peripheral glucose utilization. The positive cardiac inotropic effects of glucagon are not associated with increased peripheral resistance and may result from glucagon-induced, increased production of cyclic AMP.

490-493. The answers are: 490-C, 491-E, 492-A, 493-B. *(Martin, pp 91, 238, 295, 326.)* Clomiphene, an estrogen antagonist that was developed as a contraceptive agent, turned out to be a fertility agent in clinical trials. The drug appears to act at the pituitary gland by binding to estrogen receptors. The cells producing gonadotropins are under negative control by estrogens. When clomiphene prevents estrogen receptors from being activated, release of gonadotropins is increased.

Bromocriptine is an ergot derivative that acts like a dopaminergic agonist at the anterior pituitary gland. In normal persons, dopamine may stimulate growth hormone release. Acromegaly results from oversecretion of growth hormone; for reasons not understood, dopamine suppresses growth hormone release in some acromegalic patients. Bromocriptine is used to treat these patients because it has a longer action than dopamine.

Thyrotropin-releasing hormone (TRH) is a tripeptide released by the hypothalamus into the portal blood system connecting the hypothalamus to the anterior pituitary gland. This peptide stimulates release of both thyrotropin and prolactin. Increased triiodothyronine levels in the serum block release of both these hormones; thyrotropin release is especially sensitive to inhibition by the thyroid hormones.

Dopamine is released from the hypothalamus and acts directly upon the anterior pituitary gland to inhibit prolactin secretion. Antipsychotic drugs such as haloperidol are dopaminergic antagonists. Since dopamine tonically inhibits prolactin production, administering haloperidol causes increased prolactin release. Galactorrhea may result in both women and men.

494-496. The answers are: 494-C, 495-A, 496-E. *(Gilman, ed 6. pp 1108, 1272-1273, 1354-1355.)* Warfarin and the coumarin anticoagulants act by blocking the formation of clotting factors II, VII, IX, and X. These factors need to be carboxylated, a reaction that oxidizes the reduced form of vitamin K to an epoxide. Warfarin prevents the reduction of the vitamin K epoxide. The structural similarity between coumarin and vitamin K and the fact that vitamin K can reverse coumarin-induced hypoprothrombinemia indicate that coumarin is an antimetabolite of vitamin K.

Sulfanilamide and its derivatives (sulfonamides) prevent the synthesis of folic acid in bacteria by substrate competition with *p*-aminobenzoic acid. Bacteria that do not require folic acid, or that can use preformed folic acid, are not affected by sulfonamides.

Methotrexate serves as a folic acid antagonist and inhibits nucleic acid synthesis by blocking the enzyme dihydrofolate reductase. It is used in the treatment of acute childhood leukemia and in some cases of choriocarcinoma.

497-500. The answers are: 497-A, 498-B, 499-B, 500-E. *(Gilman, ed 6. pp 1409-1410, 1412-1413.)* Agents that can interfere directly or indirectly with the synthesis of thyroid hormones are called thyroid inhibitors. Thiocyanate, an ionic inhibitor, interferes with the capability of the thyroid to concentrate iodide by acting as a competitive inhibitor. Thiocyanate and other ionic inhibitors such as perchlorate, nitrate, and fluoborate are hydrated monovalent anions having a size similar to that of iodide.

Methimazole (Tapazole), together with thiourea, thiouracil, propylthiouracil, and other thioamides, is classified as an antithyroid drug that interferes directly with thyroid hormone synthesis. Antithyroid drugs, constituted by thioamides, aniline derivatives, and polyhydric phenols, interfere with the oxidation and incorporation of iodide into organic form and inhibit the formation of iodothyronines from the peroxidase-mediated coupling of iodotyrosines. These drugs may act by binding to peroxidase, by interacting with substrates, or by interfering with the production of hydrogen peroxide, which (in addition to oxygen) is a biologic oxidant required for the synthesis of thyroid hormones.

Iodide, most ancient of therapeutic agents for thyroid disorders, by retarding both the pinocytosis of colloid and proteolysis, inhibits the secretion of thyroid hormone. This effect is observed in euthyroid as well as hyperthyroid individuals.

Triiodothyronine is not classified as a thyroid inhibitor; it is an amino acid derivative of thyronine and results from the oxidative coupling of monoiodotyrosyl and diiodotyrosyl residues.

^{131}I, the most often used radioisotope of iodine, is rapidly absorbed by the thyroid and is deposited in follicular colloid. From the site of its deposition, ^{131}I causes fibrosis of the thyroid subsequent to pyknosis and necrosis of the follicular cells.

Bibliography

Cooper JR, Bloom FE, Roth RH: *Biochemical Basis of Neuropharmacology*, 4th ed. New York, Oxford University Press, 1982.

Craig CR, Stitzel RE (eds): *Modern Pharmacology.* Boston, Little, Brown, 1982.

Curry SH: *Drug Disposition and Pharmacokinetics*, 3rd ed. St. Louis, CV Mosby, 1981.

Doull J, Klaasen CD, Amdur MO: *Casarett and Doull's Toxicology: The Basic Science of Poisons*, 2nd ed. New York, Macmillan, 1980.

Gilman AG, et al (eds): *The Pharmacological Basis of Therapeutics*, 6th ed. New York, Macmillan, 1980.

Goth A: *Medical Pharmacology: Principles and Concepts,* 10th ed. St. Louis, CV Mosby, 1981.

Isselbacher KJ, et al (eds): *Harrison's Principles of Internal Medicine,* 9th ed. New York, McGraw-Hill, 1980.

Martin JB, Reichlin S, Brown GM: *Clinical Neuroendocrinology.* Philadelphia, FA Davis, 1977.

Pratt WB: *Chemotherapy of Infection.* New York, Oxford University Press, 1977.

Pratt WB, Ruddon RW: *The Anticancer Drugs.* New York, Oxford University Press, 1979.

Williams WJ, et al: *Hematology,* 2nd ed. New York, McGraw-Hill, 1977.